knock yourself up

# knock
# yourself up

## no man? no problem!

*A Tell-All Guide to*
*Becoming a Single Mom*

# LOUISE SLOAN

AVERY

*a member of Penguin Group (USA) Inc.*

*New York*

Published by the Penguin Group
Penguin Group (USA) Inc., 375 Hudson Street, New York, New York 10014, USA •
Penguin Group (Canada), 90 Eglinton Avenue East, Suite 700, Toronto, Ontario M4P 2Y3,
Canada (a division of Pearson Penguin Canada Inc.) • Penguin Books Ltd, 80 Strand,
London WC2R 0RL, England • Penguin Ireland, 25 St Stephen's Green, Dublin 2, Ireland (a
division of Penguin Books Ltd) • Penguin Group (Australia), 250 Camberwell Road,
Camberwell, Victoria 3124, Australia (a division of Pearson Australia Group Pty Ltd) • Penguin
Books India Pvt Ltd, 11 Community Centre, Panchsheel Park, New Delhi–110 017, India •
Penguin Group (NZ), 67 Apollo Drive, Rosedale, North Shore 0745, Auckland, New Zealand (a
division of Pearson New Zealand Ltd) • Penguin Books (South Africa) (Pty) Ltd, 24 Sturdee
Avenue, Rosebank, Johannesburg 2196, South Africa

Penguin Books Ltd, Registered Offices:
80 Strand, London WC2R 0RL, England

Most Avery books are available at special quantity discounts for bulk purchase for sales
promotions, premiums, fund-raising, and educational needs. Special books or book excerpts also
can be created to fit specific needs. For details, write Penguin Group
(USA) Inc. Special Markets, 375 Hudson Street, New York, NY 10014.

Library of Congress Cataloging-in-Publication Data

Sloan, Louise.
Knock yourself up: no man? no problem!: a tell-all guide to becoming a single mom / Louise
Sloan.
p.      cm.
Includes bibliographical references and index.
ISBN 978-1-58333-286-3
1. Artificial insemination, human—Popular works.    2. Single mothers—Popular works.
I. Title.
RG134.S57      2007                      2007028117
618.1'78—dc22

Printed in the United States of America
1   3   5   7   9   10   8   6   4   2

BOOK DESIGN BY AMANDA DEWEY

To the best of the author's knowledge, all the stories in this book are true. Most of them have not been altered at all. In some cases, however, the names have been changed, and in a few stories identifying details have been slightly altered to preserve the privacy of those involved.

Neither the publisher nor the author is engaged in rendering professional advice or services to the individual reader. The ideas, procedures, and suggestions contained in this book are not intended as a substitute for consulting with your physician. All matters regarding your health require medical supervision. Neither the author nor the publisher shall be liable or responsible for any loss or damage allegedly arising from any information or suggestion in this book.

While the author has made every effort to provide accurate telephone numbers and Internet addresses at the time of publication, neither the publisher nor the author assumes any responsibility for errors, or for changes that occur after publication. Further, the publisher does not have any control over and does not assume any responsibility for author or third-party websites or their content.

*For Scott*

# Contents

knock yourself up

# Love Makes a Family

*On the Politics of Single Motherhood
and the Purpose of This Book*

My friend Lucy became a single mother by choice—sort of," a woman told me over the tapenade at a friend's fortieth birthday party. "She wanted a kid and she was getting older, but she's from a conservative family and she really couldn't deal with what their reaction might be to her doing it alone.

"So," the woman explained, "she purposely sought out a really passive man, and within three months they were married."

"Uh," I said, channeling Dr. Phil, "how's that working for her?"

"Not so great," the woman replied. "I mean, she has a great daughter, but she has to deal with this guy who has fifty percent say in everything."

Marrying a guy only because you want kids, no other reason? It sounds a little outrageous in this day and age, but it's really as traditional as it gets. In this book, you'll meet nearly fifty women who bucked that tradition. We had children—or are thinking about having them—because we believe we have a lot to offer as moms. About the only thing we didn't have to offer our kids was a guy named Dad.

Not that we were against the idea of a dad. Most of the women in this book would love to find the right guy but, when push came to shove, decided finding a husband just wasn't their number one priority. Having a child was.

Of course, not *all* of us wanted a husband—I talked to at least one woman who prefers being single, and another who likes having boyfriends but prefers to parent on her own. Then a handful of us are gay, like me, so having our romantic partner be the father of our child was never an option. Still, most of us gay girls would have preferred to have had a child with a partner as coparent—that's certainly the case for me—but, like our straight sisters, having the child was the nonnegotiable part of the equation.

## SINGLE-PARENT FAMILY VALUES

All the women in this book pursued parenthood because we want and value family. In fact, you might say we have—dare I say it?—family values. But fifteen years after Republican Vice President Dan Quayle threw a fit about the fictional single mom on the sitcom *Murphy Brown,* creating a family without a father still sets off some right-wing folks. My original intention with this book was to start with the idea that a mature single woman with adequate resources having a baby thoughtfully on her own is an OK thing to do, and move on from there. But then I realized I should probably at least acknowledge the political and cultural debate. As I was writing the book and falling in love with my new baby boy, I watched a fairly negative talk-show segment on women who are single moms by choice and read several scathing opinion columns calling moms like me selfish, man-hating, immoral meanies. Ouch.

Actually, the single moms I have talked to seem like great parents, and before they went down this path, most spent a great deal of time thinking about—and prioritizing—the needs of their future children. Most held the idea of having a baby alone up against fairly traditional notions of family and morality and decided in the end that what they were doing was a good thing. And I think it is. I've been impressed by their courage, their thoughtfulness, and their love for their children. Their kids are lucky.

*Knock Yourself Up* does make a few apparently controversial assumptions: Single moms can be great moms. When raised in a safe, loving environment with their basic emotional and physical needs met, kids turn out OK. Being raised by a good single mom is a lot better than being brought up inside a bad marriage. Love makes a family.

As it turns out, there's a fair amount of research to back up these assumptions (for a look at some of it, see chapter 7). Still, like many of the women I talked to, I had a lot of serious concerns about choosing single motherhood. You might, too, if you're considering this path. You'll read about some of those concerns and how we worked through them. But although I discuss concerns, I offer no apologies.

## WHAT ABOUT DADS?

Like the character Murphy Brown, most of the moms in this book are "intelligent, highly paid professional wom[en]," as Quayle put it. But by raising kids on our own, are we "mocking the importance of fathers," as he opined back in 1992? I don't think so. "No man? No problem!" is part of the cheeky title of this book, and indeed not having a man was not a permanent barrier to motherhood for the women I interviewed. But for me and for most of the other women it wasn't exactly a nonissue. Most of us were very careful in considering the ramifications of having a kid who won't have a dad.

All of us have given a lot of thought to how we can give our kids the best that life has to offer, including male role models and father figures. And despite the assumptions still common to right-wing pundits, most of us value fatherhood. And men. Most women choosing single motherhood are heterosexual, and most of the ones I talked to have had plenty of suitors—they didn't go down this road because they couldn't get a date, as one negative stereotype would have it. What the straight women in this book rejected was not men or marriage—it was the idea of getting into a bad marriage, or the wrong marriage, just to have kids. Or picking any man to get pregnant by and raise a family with. In fact, many have made the decision to bear a child out of wedlock because they respect marriage too much to enter into it lightly for reasons of social and procreational expedience. Far from seeing men as unnecessary, these are women who, I'd argue, really value men and see them as equals, partners, lovers, soul mates—not as turkey basters attached to a paycheck. Finally, most of us think that having two good parents is a great thing for a kid—but we have ended up deciding that quality beats quantity where parents are concerned.

## THE POTENTIAL RISKS OF RESPECTABILITY

This brings me back to Lucy, the woman who married just to have kids in a way that would please her conservative family. There's certainly something to be said for a marriage like that, especially if both parties know what they're getting into. Lucy's kid will know her dad and will have two parents to take responsibility for her care and upbringing. That's all good. But, though marriage may be the most traditional, respectable choice, is it necessarily the most moral one in this case?

What happens when Dad discovers he's just a stud? What happens when Mom decides she maybe doesn't want to spend the rest of her life shackled to that random guy? What happens when their daughter realizes that Mom and Dad aren't a love match? That, for Mom, Dad was just sperm, a paycheck, and a mantle of respectability? It all could go relatively well. But it could be a tinderbox, a recipe for upheaval and pain. Marriage can be a wonderful thing if entered into for the right reasons, and it can be a terrific structure within which to raise a family. But it isn't a magic wand that will ensure safety and happiness. This mom's bid for stability and respectability could easily end up resulting in an unhappy, unstable environment for her kid.

## THE NEW BREED OF SINGLE MOMS

The well-being of their kids was the main concern of most of the moms in this book. That's probably a big concern for you, too, if you're considering parenting alone. Will the kids be OK? It's a good question. Single motherhood gets a bad rap. Deservedly so, it seems. There are statistics galore about how bad it is for the children, how they tend to drop out of high school, turn to crime, use drugs, and otherwise suffer the consequences. But those grim statistics are about single teen moms without adequate financial, educational, or community resources. The stats are also about divorced moms who thought they were all set with a husband, then find they can't manage as well after the divorce, raising angry, hurt kids while they are alone and experiencing a sudden drop in income and a dramatic shift in lifestyle. I could suggest that blaming this entirely on the moms is not the way to go, but that's another book.

2

The women in this book constitute another, newer set of single moms, a set that hasn't been taken into account by most studies: educated adult women, usually over thirty, who want to have kids and who have the resources to do it alone. Not that we are all rich—some are, but others are far from it. But if not rich in cash, we generally have an adequate amount. More important, we have the personal resources to pull off parenthood, to figure things out if times get tough, to make sure the kids are OK. In researching this book, I talked to more than fifty single moms or aspiring single moms from all over the country and listened in to the discussions of hundreds of others in meetings and Internet discussion groups. Most of us decided on single motherhood after much thought and as a real choice—not because we literally had no other options. And, unlike Murphy Brown, who decided to continue rather than abort her accidental pregnancy, we got pregnant on purpose.

## WHAT ABOUT ADOPTION?

*Knock Yourself Up* is specifically about single women who, like me, decided they wanted to bear their own biological child. "Isn't that selfish?" I've been asked. Maybe it is—though I am not sure *selfish* is the right word for choosing to take complete responsibility for another person's care for eighteen-plus years. But if it is selfish, it's a primal selfishness, one that's shared by just about everybody. Adoption is the better thing for anyone to do, single or married. And some of the moms in this book have adopted, in addition to having biological children. But adoption is a different path with its own issues and complications. This book is about single women who not only want to raise a child but who, like so many other women, want the messy, scary, beautiful, animal experience of having a baby grow inside them, of giving birth, of knowing another human being from the moment of conception, and of having a deeply physical, biological connection to a child.

## SO, WHAT KIND OF BOOK IS THIS?

*Knock Yourself Up* is a girlfriends' guide, subjective as hell. (A clink of the Cosmopolitan glass to Vicki Iovine, author of *The Girlfriends' Guide to Pregnancy* and queen of the *Girlfriends' Guide* publishing empire, no relation to this book.) There are already two excellent how-to books on choosing single motherhood, based on sound psychology and reams of research: the now classic *Single Mothers by Choice*, first published in 1994 by psychotherapist and single mom Jane Mattes, and the newer, breathtakingly thorough *Choosing Single Motherhood: The Thinking Woman's Guide*, by Mikki Morrissette, a single mom of two. They'll tell you exactly what you should do, laying out the issues step by step.

This is a different kind of book. Though I brought in some experts to help elucidate a few of the thornier issues, *Knock Yourself Up* is generally light on research and heavy on anecdotes, covering both the serious and the silly. Not everyone has as many crazy capers on the way to single motherhood as I did, though most women do find something to chuckle about as they go to absurd lengths and often great expense to do something that's supposed to be so natural and come so easily.

On the warm, fuzzy side of things, many single moms by choice find, as I did, that most people—even conservative grandparents-to-be and small-town strangers—turn out to be surprisingly supportive of the decision once you give them a chance. But as heartwarming or funny as choosing single motherhood can sometimes be, it can also be hard, heartbreaking, and lonely. When I was going through it, there wasn't anything out there to give me the real dirt on what it's like, physically and emotionally, to go through this process as a single woman. It's different for everyone, to be sure. But it's my hope that by sharing my experience and the experiences of many others, you'll get a clearer picture of what might lie ahead, both good and bad. Most of all, I hope reading this book will be like talking to a group of friends who have been there before you—helping you feel that, even though you may be going it alone, you're in good company.

## WHO ARE THE WOMEN IN THIS BOOK?

Just like in many real friendships, my "girlfriends" and I have had totally different experiences. In fact, on some points, we completely disagree. And that's precisely the point. *Knock Yourself Up* is meant to be a lively support group in text form, offering a diversity of perspectives. Of the forty-three women I interviewed at length for the book, most are members of the group Single Mothers by Choice who answered a call I placed on their online bulletin board. Other than that, these moms and moms-to-be are all over the map—literally. I spoke to a lot of women in New York and California—the usual suspects for "alternative" choices—but also in Ohio, Kansas, Texas, Georgia, Utah, New Mexico, New Jersey, Michigan, Colorado, Maryland, Virginia, Maine, Pennsylvania, New Hampshire, Wisconsin, Massachusetts, and Canada. (I could have talked to women in Australia, England, and Israel, but I didn't want to pay the phone bills!)

The women in *Knock Yourself Up* are also fairly diverse in terms of race, ethnicity, and sexual orientation. Five of the women I interviewed are Black, one is both Native American and African-American, and one is both Puerto Rican and Filipina; the other thirty-six are white. My numbers of Black, white, and Asian interviewees are roughly in proportion to the percentages of those groups in the general population. I am not sure why I didn't get more Latina women responding to my interview requests. I know they are out there; perhaps they just weren't members of the groups through which I sought interview subjects or they didn't feel comfortable sharing their stories with me. Lisa M., the Puerto Rican–Filipina woman I interviewed, said that she went to a single mom's support group meeting for a while but quickly dropped out. "I stopped going because there was no one who looked like me. I just didn't fit in." As for sexual orientation, the majority—thirty-seven—of the women I interviewed are straight. Six are gay.

One thing most of the moms in the book do have in common is that they are middle-class. The vast majority are college-educated women with white-collar jobs, though I spoke to a few with other educational backgrounds and to some who are artists or have careers in the service industry. I didn't ask anyone to disclose her salary, but I heard numbers ranging from $20,000 (what one single mom made the year she was pregnant) to $250,000. I'd guess most make somewhere between $50,000 and $100,000.

Now, there are plenty of single women who decide to be solo parents for the same reasons as the women here but who do not have the same kind of educational background and income level. With enough determination and community support, their kids can do fine, too. In fact, a 2004 multiethnic Cornell University study found that the kids of educated, able moms tend to do well even if they're living below the poverty line. There are some who basically position child rearing as a middle-class privilege, something that's OK only if you have a certain amount of money. That's not right, but the reality is that without certain educational, financial, and community resources, raising kids alone can be a lot harder, and those kids are more likely to represent the grim single-mom statistics. This book specifically deals with the smaller segment of single mothers who have incomes that make it possible (though not always easy) to support a family.

In any case, while my sample is neither scientific nor comprehensive, there's a fairly wide range of experience represented by the women I talked to. I hope that reading our stories will give you a feel for what choosing to be a single mom is *really like*—and what it might be like for you.

And why it might *not* be for you. I hope this book will help you if you really want to be a mom, but I also hope it might dissuade you if you feel you *should* be a mom. Single motherhood is still considered a radical choice in mainstream America, particularly among middle-class white women, but choosing *not* to be a mom is probably considered the strangest choice of all. That's too bad. There are a million excellent reasons not to have kids, starting with the best one of all: "I don't want to." Likewise, there are a million good reasons to have kids, but there are some terrible ones as well. Like "everyone else does," or "my parents are pressuring me for a grandchild," or "I don't feel like I'll be a real woman until I'm a mom." Or, how can we forget, the number one bad reason to get into any relationship: "I'm miserable and lonely, and a child (boyfriend/girlfriend/cupcake/cigarette/martini) will solve all those problems."

Since I live in New York City, I don't have a car. This means I have nowhere to put bumper stickers—which may be why I seem to feel compelled to plaster them all over this author's note. I already pasted one in here earlier: Love Makes a Family. So I'll end with another: Every Child a Wanted Child.

As my bumper stickers suggest, I am what you might call a liberal. Some of the other moms in this book would call themselves conservative. I live in the Big Apple, while many of the other moms live in Middle America. I'm gay, and most of the women I talked to are straight. But one thing that definitely unites me and all of my single-mama "girlfriends" across the country, besides the fact that we tend to be pretty self-confident and independent, is that we really, really, really wanted our children. And that, I hope we can all agree, is a good thing.

# Introduction:
# How I Knocked
# Myself Up

t was Labor Day weekend. I'd had the semen tank delivered to my mom's
summer house in Kennebunkport, down the road from the Bushes. The
ovulation test stick said it was time. So, after breakfast, I collected what
I needed from the kitchen—mixing bowl and bag for thawing the vials,
bright yellow dishwashing gloves as protection against the subzero liquid
nitrogen—and told my mother it was time to "baste" (as in turkey). She
looked at me as if I'd just told her I was going to run upstairs to give myself
an enema. Clearly I'd lost perspective, expecting my seventy-year-old conservative Republican Southern mama to be totally cool with having a
stranger's frozen sperm FedExed to her front porch, for the purpose of knocking up her single, forty-one-year-old lesbian daughter.

How did I get to this point? It started thirteen years earlier, when I
dragged my then-partner, Joan, to a six-week gay and lesbian parenting sem-
inar in San Francisco, where we lived at the time. We learned about the
legal, medical, and logistical issues around having kids outside a heterosexual marriage, then joined a monthly brunch group of gays considering parenthood. Twenty men and women would gather in someone's living room
in Berkeley or Bernal Heights and, over coffee and a potluck, discuss their
various child-rearing dreams. Mine was to find a friend willing to be both the

donor and an uncle figure to the kid. Joan and I would then each bear a child, performing the inseminations at home, by candlelight, and we'd all live happily ever after. Right.

Ten years and three breakups later, I was thirty-eight, single, living in Manhattan, and no closer to motherhood. I joined another group: Single Lesbians Considering Parenthood. We were *all* thirty-eight. This being the big city, there was neither potluck nor living room. Twelve of us sat around a grim conference table at the gay community center and talked about the terrors of single motherhood, and the logistics, too: adoption versus pregnancy, known donors versus sperm banks. Having grown up without a dad (he died before I was two), I really wanted a known donor—a friend. Three years later, after agonizing and asking male friends, and various other delays, I was all set to start. Age forty-one. Single. Anonymous donor sperm. At the doctor's office. The inverse of my dream, but my bio clock was sounding more like a car alarm.

## HOLIDAYS ON ICE

The first intrauterine insemination didn't take. And my doctor's office was closed for the Labor Day holiday, when I'd next be ripe. I'd have to skip a month or do it the old-fashioned turkey-baster way. I chose the baster. Or, more accurately, the one-milliliter tuberculin syringe (without a needle, of course!), which is the way women are basted these days.

Up in the attic of my mother's summer cottage, in a little blue-and-white bedroom overlooking the ocean, I prepared to do the deed. When I carefully unscrewed the two little plastic vials (they were two for one, since the donor's sperm count was low on that deposit day—"Sweetie, your dad was on sale!"), the excited little containers, pressurized from their plane ride from California, exploded all over my fingers. This was *way* more like the real thing than what happened in the doctor's office.

I lay flat for the prescribed two hours, flipping myself around like a rotisserie chicken (also suggested for best results), looking out the window at the ocean and reading my sister's latest Danielle Steel novel. My cell phone rang and it was, ironically, one of my male friends who'd said no to donorhood. We chatted while I basted. I did the whole thing again the next morning. Like good WASPs, my family did not speak of it.

When it didn't take, it was back to the doctor's office. Three months and three tries later, still no dice. My next fertile holiday was Christmas—I was due to ovulate on Boxing Day. I called the sperm bank in San Francisco and ordered a tank to go to my mom's again, this time to her home in Richmond, Virginia. It would arrive, via second-day air, on Christmas Eve.

Christmas Eve morning broke and my ovulation test stick turned, two days early. I had to inseminate as soon as possible or I'd miss my egg's window of fertility. I wrapped presents. I paced. I waited. I refused to leave the house to run helpful errands for my mom. We fought about the five o'clock church service—I said I had to wait for FedEx. Never came. My sister said she'd heard they were doing some deliveries Christmas Day. So I stayed home again, my egg's time clock about to sound its final alarm, missing Christmas Day service, too, for the first time ever.

At last, on Saturday, the day after Christmas, I got some answers from FedEx. Snowstorms in the Midwest. The tank was in the holding area at the Oakland airport. It would arrive Tuesday, way too late to get me pregnant. I said it actually now had to go back to San Francisco. "Sorry," the agent said. "It's already staged for delivery." Lover boy had to travel six thousand miles round-trip just to get back across the San Francisco Bay. Worse, he would arrive on the East Coast on his last breath of liquid nitrogen.

I sprang into gear, arranging to have the tank held at FedEx so I could pick it up first thing, and finding a welding-supply store that would refill it with nitrogen so the sperm wouldn't spoil. Tuesday morning, I drove out to FedEx, located on Studley Road, no lie. I gave my name, mentioning that my package had been delayed, and the clerk went back to find it. As she lugged the tank up to the counter, she said, loudly, in a thick, chirpy Southern accent, "Ah swear, it's always you semen people who get the late deliveries!" Then she launched into a funny story about a veterinarian. Right. I'm breeding champion Chihuahuas. I guess not much else arrives in tanks like that. I smiled and hurried out the door, sticking my semen into the huge backseat of my mother's wood-grained station wagon. The welding guys filled the tank, twice (first time it wasn't closed properly and started hissing in the backseat like a bomb), and it was back to the sperm bank's San Fran deep freeze for my little swimmers.

Obviously, that try yielded nothing. Meanwhile, I called the sperm bank to get Don Juan's pregnancy stats, and they were grim. He was tall, dark-haired, blue-eyed, and handsome, but he wasn't getting anyone pregnant. I started to suspect I was using blanks. My next window would open on Groundhog Day. I decided to do it both at home and at the doc's, for extra luck. I was seeing someone, so I asked her if she would help. Science experiment complete, we forgot ourselves, and, well—afterward, I was worried that I may have knocked *her* up (but more on that later). Crazy in love, I was secretly excited. Aloud, I apologized profusely and pledged full child support. Alas, Mr. Blanks didn't do it for either of us. I gave up on the guy. Then the girl ditched me.

In April, Donor Number Two, a tall, handsome, green-eyed actor ("Favorite color: blue. Favorite pet: dogs"), got me pregnant on his second try. Sadly, on Memorial Day weekend, back in K'port again, I miscarried. It was my littlest niece's first birthday. Leah and Tyler, ages six and eight, didn't understand why Aunt Weeze didn't want to jump on the trampoline. At least there was no pain, and it was nice to be surrounded by family.

Two failed tries later, and it was Labor Day again. Time for my annual "inseminate at Mom's summer house" tradition. My tank arrived a day late due to Hurricane Katrina, but the test stick kept not turning. By Friday, I wondered if I was just not going to ovulate that month, and I realized the tank was going to run out of nitrogen by Sunday. It was off to Advantage Gases and Tools, welding suppliers for southernmost Maine.

The burly middle-aged guys behind the counter were nice, though my request was an unusual one for them. "This medical?" the shorter one asked. "Yeah," I said, without elaboration. He took it into the back to fill it up, while his tall, equally burly colleague futzed with the computer, trying to figure out how to code the sale of a small amount of nitrogen.

We waited, and finally the guy at the computer asked, "So—what you using it for?" I figured why not tell the truth, but I wanted to word it delicately. "I'm, uh, trying to get pregnant." The big guy got flustered at first, then confided: "My wife and I didn't have to go the fertility route," he said, "but we lost three before we had our first son." This huge welding-supply salesman and I then had a sweet conversation about the kids in our lives.

At last, Short Guy came out from the back, carrying the tank, with a funny expression on his face. "So—you got horses or something?" His colleague and I cracked up. "You *don't* wanna know!" said Tall Guy in his thick Maine accent.

By the Sunday before Labor Day, my egg was finally ready. Green Eyes and I did it the turberculin way in my sweet attic bedroom overlooking the

sea. This time, as I was stretched out in my nightgown on the bed, basting—actually I was flat on my stomach with my chin on my laptop, typing a work e-mail—my mom came up with some Concord grapes to chat. The empty inch-long plastic vial was next to me on the sheet I'd laid over the bedspread, so I held it up and said, "I should introduce you to Dad." My mom laughed. "Nice to meet ya, Dad," she said. Then my youngest sister yelled, "Knock knock," and came in, wanting to talk about her new house. Mom interrupted: "Louise, you should introduce Caroline to Dad." I picked up the vial again. "Caroline, this is Dad. Dad, Caroline." My insemination was turning out to be a family-values event.

That afternoon, I had a three-and-a-half-hour drive to The Forks, Maine (population: thirty-five), to meet a couple of friends for a white-water rafting trip. I had Mom take a picture of me strapping "Dad" in his nitrogen tank into the backseat with the seat belt. "Louise and Dad go rafting." The next insemination (the standard is to do two in a row each month) was a group effort. I'd forgotten the syringe, so Mae, Susan, and I went into Girl Scout mode, crafting a substitute using available objects in our small log cabin in the woods: a thin plastic bag and a cardboard tampon applicator. Rustic—but it worked. Next morning, as I floated in my life preserver in the cold water of the Kennebec River's "swimmer's rapids," it occurred to me that I may not be optimizing conception. But it sure was fun.

I would love to say that was the time Green Eyes got me pregnant again. In fact, conception happened about a month later, September 30, at the doctor's office. "Accomplished easily with a long Peterson and a Tomcat," my patient chart says, referring to the type of speculum and catheter the doctor used. Sounds like WWII artillery. But in my heart, my son was conceived on Labor Day in Kennebunkport and The Forks, surrounded by my lesbian friends and my loving Republican family.

# Oops! I Forgot to Have a Baby!

## *Deciding to Go It Alone*

Have a baby solo? Some women really don't sweat it. Take Marcy, a Navy officer stationed in Georgia. Her decision to become a single mother was, as befits a military officer, fairly cut-and-dried: a cost-benefit analysis. She was thirty-three—fertilitywise, that's getting up there. Because of military rules about fraternizing with inferiors, "my available pool of who to date was cut down to one person—and I dated him!" the blond-haired, dimpled mom recalls, laughing. Besides, dating just wasn't all that much fun anymore. "I was tired of guys pretending to be someone they are not, or wanting me to pretend to be something I'm not," she says. "It just seemed like the single guys my age were single for a reason. Plus, I looked around and everyone I knew was married and had kids. And I realized I wanted to be a mother more than I wanted to be a wife."

Decision made, no angst, no hand-wringing. Marcy ordered up some sperm, went to her gynecologist, and got herself pregnant.

"For me it was all logistics," says Ellen, a long-haired, light-skinned African-American lawyer in Washington, D.C., who has two daughters by anonymous donor insemination. When she realized becoming a single mom was an option, her main questions were practical ones: "Can I afford this, do I have the time, do I have the right job for this?

"It wasn't until I was pregnant that I heard about the group Single Mothers by Choice," she said. The two-thousand-member organization has an online community of nearly a thousand "thinkers," who often spend years sweating it out in cyberspace before they take the next step.

Oh, shit, Ellen thought, should I have thought more deeply about this?

Same story, more or less, for Debrah, a surgeon in Toronto, who applied to her personal life the same logic she'd used to maintain her successful medical career. "There comes a point when you have to sit down and assess what your goals are. Then you have to take concrete steps." So she did some research, talked to some other single moms, and soon enough had a baby boy. Clearheaded. Logical. Adult.

This was not me.

When I think about my willingness to become a single parent, a panel from cartoonist Eric Orner's *The Mostly Unfabulous Social Life of Ethan Green* comes to mind. It's in a strip about leaving the beach at the end of a summer weekend, done according to the Five Stages of Grief, from Elisabeth Kübler-Ross's famous book *On Death and Dying*. In the panel labeled Depression (stage four), it's Sunday, and Ethan, a gay man in his late twenties, is still out in the ocean in Provincetown. Work starts early Monday morning in Boston, a two-and-a-half-hour drive away.

"Ethan," one of his older drag-queen friends says, maternally, "it's Sunday noon, cupcake, shouldn't you be heading back to the city?"

"No no no no no no no," says Ethan, curled in fetal position, clinging to his inflatable raft.

That's exactly how I felt about single motherhood.

I was ready for kids at age twenty-eight, and I was well aware that women's fertility really starts to plummet at thirty-five. Even if I hadn't been aware, my harshly proactive doctor would have put me on notice. When I went in for my physical the year I turned thirty-five, she asked me if I wanted kids. When I said yes, she looked at me sternly and snapped, "Well, you're not getting any younger!"

Thanks for the news flash, I thought. What kind of idiot does she think I am?

I was a romantic, procrastinating idiot, to be exact. I did not want to give up the dream of having the partner first, and then the baby. That dream was not only what I wanted, but also what I wanted for my child. I knew I'd be a great mom, with a lot to give. But I wanted my kid to have two parents—

a luxury I did not have myself, since my dad died when I was very young. In fact, I wanted there to be *three* parents: two mommies and a noncustodial dad, my lesbian version of the white-picket-fence dream. So, despite a perfectly clear intellectual understanding of the fertility issues involved, it took me to age thirty-eight before I seriously started thinking about single motherhood, and I had to be dragged into it kicking and screaming by my biological clock.

Not only did I kick and scream, but I worried—no, agonized—in exhaustive detail, about every single thing you could possibly worry about. Starting with the big one: Was it fair to the child to have only one parent and no dad? Month after hideous month, I spun out elaborate scenarios of my future fifteen-year-old's painful psychological struggle with his or her unusual birth circumstances, and I'd cry for him. Or her. Sure, everything I'd ever read about alternative families with donor dads indicated that the kids do just fine—studies show that most have a surprising lack of angst, or even interest, regarding their unusual roots (for more on that, see Chapter 7). But try telling that to the black hole of worry that had taken up residence in my psyche, sucking all possible positive outcomes into oblivion.

When I wasn't keening over my future child's imaginary angst, I worried about myself. Was it fair to *me* to become a single parent? Could I even do it? Would I die of loneliness? Would I become this crazy overinvolved mom with nothing else in my life? Would I never have a romantic life again? What if I can't afford it? What if the child turns out to be seriously handicapped? What if I don't sleep for ten years?

One of the women I interviewed for this book put it perfectly: "When I first made the decision, I'd go to bed and worry about what I'd cook for my five-year-old." Well, not that it's a competition, but I think I win. I worried more than any of the women I've ever spoken to, and I procrastinated more than most, though maybe some of them just weren't 'fessing up. By the time I got my act together, I was forty-one and could easily have missed my fertility window. I was lucky.

Min, an artist and teacher in New York City, with long auburn hair and a breathy, girlish voice, had similarly cold feet. She started thinking about single motherhood in her midthirties and attended support groups about once a year for a couple years, but she could not bring herself to act. "The whole thought of conceiving without a partner and without love was not appealing to me," she says. "Then when I started calling around to cryobanks—

that freaked me out. Choosing sperm, picking the father of your child in this way, freaked me out." Plus, she says, "I really enjoy having sex." So the antiseptic process of insemination at a doctor's office was not a big draw. "It was a long process for me to get over each one of these hurdles," Min says. "That delayed me for a few years." At last, there was a sudden shift in her attitude. "Something just clicked inside me and there was no hesitation." Unfortunately, Min, who's now forty-two and trying to get pregnant but facing fertility problems, is finding that she may have delayed for so long that achieving pregnancy will turn out to be wildly expensive—or impossible.

Some women have an equally hard time giving up the dream, but start thinking about it at a more sensible age. Take Shannon, a veterinary technician who lives outside Los Angeles with her dog, five cats, and a guinea pig. "I was a 'thinker' for ten years before I finally bit the bullet," she says. At twenty-five, she had "maternal longings," but was still "looking for Mr. Right or Mr. Good Enough." Around age thirty she realized she better come up with Plan B. "I kept putting it off and hoping that Plan A would work," she says, "but around my thirty-fourth birthday I realized I was reaching the point of now or never." For Shannon, pursuing single motherhood was mostly a clearheaded financial decision. "I knew if I kept waiting, I'd be more likely to have fertility problems, and that wouldn't work out for me financially." But the choice had its mystical elements, too. Shannon looked for a sign that what she was doing was right. "I had a friend do a tarot reading for me about a decision I had to make," she says. "I didn't tell her what it was." The cards promised her heartbreak (the Three of Swords) if she did not proceed with her plans and "the beginning of a joyful enterprise" (the Ace of Cups) if she did. The final card that came up as the "advice of the tarot" was Death, which represents change and transformation, Shannon says. "The tarot was telling me to let go of something that was holding me back—in this case, me clinging to the 'fantasy' of first finding Mr. Right, then starting a family. The cards pointed me toward becoming a SMC [single mother by choice]. So that kind of gave me the push," she says, laughing at the idea of having brought superstition into such a serious decision.

Cheri, who works for an ad agency in Kansas, had had single motherhood as Plan B in mind for a long time. "When I was seventeen," she remembers, "I told my high school boyfriend that if I wasn't married by thirty, I'd have a child on my own." So naturally, when she turned thirty, Cheri thought about it. For a minute. "I just wasn't ready," she says. But by age thirty-four, she decided she'd better get busy. "I felt like I was in a really good place in my career and I had a good support system," she says. "I gave one last relationship my best effort, and that didn't work, for whatever reason. I decided it was time."

Still, Cheri "kind of eased into it," she says. She bought the book *Single Mothers by Choice*. She talked it over with her parents: "They were good sounding boards." She thought through insemination versus adoption. She consolidated her debt. Then she hit what was, for her, the hardest question: Did this mean she'd never marry? "That was the last hurdle before becoming a single mother by choice. Somehow in my head, making that choice meant being single forever," Cheri says.

"I decided it didn't mean that," she says, simply. Indeed it did not. Cheri is now the happy single mom of a two-year-old son—and she's dating.

Jenny, an artist and teacher living in New York City, started thinking about it at age thirty-three, when she complained to her therapist about a friend who seemed to be living an impossibly charmed life. The friend had wanted to get married before she was thirty, and presto, she got back in touch with her high school sweetheart and they were married shortly after. Jenny's friend had her next few years all planned out: world travel, then a baby. What was it, exactly, that was making Jenny so jealous about her friend, the therapist wanted to know.

"I just hate it that she knows when she's going to have a kid."

Well, what about Jenny? When did *she* want to have a kid?

"I don't know, probably when I'm thirty-six," Jenny replied.

"So start getting curious about how it's going to happen," the therapist said.

"I can't, I'm not even dating anyone right now," Jenny said. She didn't see how she'd have time to get into a solid relationship, much less get married and start a family in three years, with some guy she hadn't even met.

"If you can't get serious about when it's going to happen, it's not going to happen," the therapist warned.

Jenny was still resistant to even thinking about it, but after that conversation she says she did find herself "getting curious" about how she could have a baby on the timetable she wanted. Slowly but surely, she talked to people and examined her own feelings. Now, at thirty-six, Jenny, a tall, easy-going, pretty woman with dark, wavy hair and a warm smile, is in her second trimester of a healthy pregnancy. The sequence of events isn't the way she originally hoped it would be—true love, marriage, baby—but she decided

"I just need to think about it in a different order." And in the meantime, she is not letting her childbearing dreams pass her by.

For Charlene, an educational consultant in Chicago, it was her gynecologist who gave her the push. "I had planned to adopt, because I'm African-American. I knew there were so many children who needed families." But working in the public schools with a lot of adopted children, Charlene realized that the older, needy kids she wanted to adopt would require more of her than she felt she could give as a single parent. Then, at age thirty-nine, during a routine checkup, her doctor reminded her of the simple biological fact: "If you want to have kids, you need to have them." As in, now. Charlene researched single motherhood and asked herself, "Do I really want to have a baby or do I want to adopt?" And she came to a realization: "Even if I adopted, I always wanted to carry a child. I just couldn't miss it."

## TAKING THE "DADDY" OUT OF DATING

As Cheri, the Kansas ad executive, has found, dating can work out, post-baby. But for most women I've spoken to, there came a point, prebaby, where their biological clocks became serious dating hazards.

"As I got closer to thirty-five, dating got panicky," says Nicole, a marketing executive based in Toronto, who was trying everything—setups from friends, bookstores, online dating, you name it—in her quest to meet Mr. Right. "As that clock started ticking, each time a date didn't go well I'd feel a huge loss. It was all about the baby—and as much as I tried not to show those feelings on a date, I'm sure they came through loud and clear."

Jamie, an energetic, attractive children's book buyer in New York City, felt the same. "I was trying too hard to make every relationship something serious; after three dates, usually the guy would bail," she says. "I realized I was dating to find a husband and father to my child, and that's why it wasn't working." Now that she's decided to get pregnant as a single woman, she feels in a healthier position for dating. "I still want to meet somebody, but this has taken the pressure off."

Ellen, the lawyer in D.C., came to the single-motherhood crossroads after another relationship ended. The breakup came at about the point where she'd been asking herself, "Where is this going, can I have kids with this guy?" She was disgusted.

"Why should I settle for something like this?" she asked herself. "I decided to stop wasting my time with ridiculous relationships; stop trying to make them more than they are just because I want to get married and have children."

Melissa, a corporate meeting planner in New York City with ash-blond hair and a decisive manner, *was* married—and she thought she and her husband had agreed to have kids. When, five years later, it became clear he didn't want them, Melissa divorced him. "I was willing to compromise on a lot of things, but not that," she says. But at thirty-four, newly single, and craving kids, she brought a crazy intensity to the dating scene. Going out on a date, she was single-minded: "How can I get this man to fall in love with me and marry me and have children with me?" Melissa says, laughing. "That was all I cared about." Needless to say, desperation dating wasn't working too well. At last, Melissa came up with a single-motherhood plan and set the plan in motion. Perhaps not coincidentally, the next thing she knew, she had a boyfriend. For Melissa, the bottom line was a simple one: "I realized the things I regretted most in my life were the things I had chosen not to do."

The biological clock can screw up dating even if you're not looking for a partner who can get you pregnant. Liz, a nonprofit manager in New York City who is now the single mom of three-year-old twins, had the same story so many other women do. When she hit her midthirties, she realized, "I was pushing the issue about having a kid with people who were clearly not the right people for me." Since Liz is a lesbian, a donor dad was always going to be part of the picture. But she was looking for a coparent. "Whether you're gay or straight you operate the same way," Liz says. "If you're a woman and you're wanting to have a child, it becomes impossible at some point to date without that being your priority." Finally, around age thirty-six, Liz concluded that with her baby-centered mind-set "it was impossible to get into a relationship that was healthy," and decided to focus entirely on what had clearly become her number one priority anyway—having a kid.

## GRAPPLING WITH NEW GENDER ROLES

Most of the single moms I've spoken to were raised, as I was, with traditional expectations of marriage and family, but have come of childbearing age at a time when those institutions are undergoing a major shift.

Women are actually starting to come closer to equality in the workplace, and marriage has become less of an economic and social necessity. It's a shift that's been going on for a while, one that has spawned a lot of angry best sellers as men and women try to figure it all out: there's *The Second Shift*, sociologist Arlie Hochschild's 1989 classic about how working wives are still doing all the housework; more recently, *Perfect Madness: Motherhood in the Age of Anxiety*, an angry postfeminist manifesto about trying to be supermom, and *The Mommy Wars*, about working moms versus stay-at-home moms; and, more colorfully and perhaps more to the point, the companion anthologies *The Bitch in the House* and *The Bastard on the Couch*, which consist, basically, of a bunch of the one expletive venting about a bunch of the other.

As a result of all this upheaval, as the *New York Times* reported in January 2007, 51 percent of American women are living without a spouse. We've thrown out the old system because it wasn't working, but we haven't figured out a new way. In the meantime, should half of all American women give up on ever having kids? The women in this book think not.

The women I interviewed are, not surprisingly, a strong-willed, fairly independent bunch. "Like a lot of women, I put my career first," says Marcy, now the thirty-six-year-old single mom of a two-and-a-half-year-old son. "And I don't really regret it. I had the opportunity to do a lot of great things I wouldn't have been able to do with a child." Still, like the struggling subjects of all those books, most still had certain dreams and expectations that were more closely aligned with fifties sitcoms than with twenty-first-century social shifts. The struggle still goes on for most of us. We've seen what taking on a domestic, dependent role can do to a woman, what settling into a perfunctory marriage can do to the two poor souls involved and how damaging it can be for the children. Yet having a child alone is not most women's childhood dream, and becoming a single mom is, for most women, a mother of a compromise. But one thing this younger generation of working women is not willing to do is to make the compromise often made by the women before them, who achieved career success but with the price tag of childlessness.

"I expected to be married at twenty-three and have six kids by the time I was thirty," says Nina, a project manager from Baltimore. She majored in theater in college, and her plan was to become an enlightened housewife: "I'll get married to someone who makes a decent living and I'll volunteer and have a theater company on the side," she added. Instead, she is startled to find that she has practically become the man she'd wanted to marry: "I made my way up in the business world, I had a baby on my own, and I do theater on the side."

Even so, Nina says she was holding on to the dream of finding a man, falling in love, getting married, and then having children. She was pushed into single motherhood for medical reasons—she had to have a hysterectomy as a precaution against cancer, and needed to have a baby quickly before the operation or give up on biological parenthood. But she finds that her decision to have a child alone puts her in what feels like a better position for finding a mate and fulfilling the heart of her dreams. "It kind of takes the pressure off," she says. "I can meet people for who they are and whether we're a good match or not."

Nicole, the marketing executive from Toronto, finds herself in waters similarly uncharted by her childhood expectations: "I never imagined I'd be this career person with a job I love, working for a company I love," she says. But this success in the public sphere isn't quite satisfying enough. Neither is her single lifestyle, full and happy as it is. "I travel on my own, I backpack, I've got so many great things going for me," Nicole says. (Indeed she does. At my request, she sent me a picture of herself. In the photo, Nicole—a strikingly attractive woman with long dark hair, olive skin, and an engaging smile—is face-to-face with a camel on one of her many trips. The image looks like something out of an *Elle* magazine fashion spread. "But as great as all that is, it has never made me want to have a child less." And, she adds, she's worked for a lot of very successful older women—women who have neither married nor had kids.

"They travel, they own their own homes," Nicole says. "But as great as everything looks, there is a lonely, sad feeling about them. And I could see that if I didn't do something about this, that was the road I would go down." While the "lonely, sad feeling" may be a projection on Nicole's end—many women happily choose to be childfree—it is true that for others, being childfree was not a real choice.

Despite the gains in women's workplace equality, some things haven't changed all that much. The business world has not adjusted its policies, expectations, and practices to allow workers of both genders to balance career and family. Some of the single moms I have spoken to have been able to maintain successful careers and have a baby. But many have shifted onto more of a mommy track—sometimes by choice, sometimes not. And despite all the talk about Mom and apple pie, American business isn't exactly family friendly. Business still operates the way it did when most families were single-earner, male-headed households, where the mom stayed home and cared for the kids and the dad worked so hard he never saw them. The result is that moms generally have to downgrade their careers, and dads are generally deprived of being real, hands-on parents. It's a scenario that's bad for everyone, in my opinion: men, women, and children.

Anne, a writer and Web-marketing manager from California who decided to become a single mom after already having had a kid within a relationship, feels grateful that she didn't have to make the decision to be a single mom because of the ticking biological clock, a decision she sees friends of hers grappling with now. "You have to give up a career, or at least career advancement," she says. "It's this huge sacrifice, a huge, huge decision. I know a lot of women who struggle with it, and it's easier not to take action than to take action. There's always, like, one hundred reasons not to do it. But I wonder, in twenty years—those women who didn't have kids, are they going to regret it, or are they going to have satisfaction with where their careers have taken them?"

Many women who have chosen single motherhood are "reluctant revolutionaries," as Wellesley sociologist Rosanna Hertz calls them in her book *Single by Chance, Mothers by Choice*. These single moms long for something closer to the traditional family but are unwilling to wait for Prince Charming forever. Some simply become more pragmatic with age and experience: "If you've been married once, the fairy tale aspect of that fades," says Debrah. It's not just limited to one's own experience. "I've seen so many of my friends in marriages that are fucking disasters," says Jenny, nineteen weeks pregnant. "I realized I could do worse than to do this on my own."

Some women actually embrace the revolution, however, and are absolutely thrilled to be living in an age where the traditions are more easily bypassed. Though their views may seem unusual or even offensive, they may just be the canaries in the coal mine of a society that's still having a lot of trouble figuring out how romantic love and family life can work with equality of the sexes. Kimberley, a fiery single mom from Portland, Maine, who talks almost faster than my slow Southern ears can listen, is one of them. "I adore men!" she says. "But I never felt that dying urge to get married." Still, to have a baby, she says, "I'd been so conditioned to think the next step was to find a man." When she came to the idea of having a kid alone and realized it was both doable and at least borderline acceptable, it was an "I could've had a V8!" moment for her. "I couldn't believe that I'd never thought of this before," Kimberley says, gushing. "We're so lucky!"

Eva, a psychotherapist in New York who is trying to conceive, feels a bit more mixed about it. Part of her does hold on to the typical fantasy of having kids within a love relationship. But Eva, who has short streaked-blond hair and striking light blue eyes, was raised in Israel under Orthodox Judaism. In that tradition, if you're a woman, she says, there are many restrictions. For example, she says, "You're not allowed to sing in front of a man." Eva has gone through a lot to distance herself from all that, and though she hopes for a partner, she also holds her independence very dear, a quality she shares with some others who have chosen single motherhood. "There's a reason I'm single," she says. "Relationships involve a lot of compromise, and I want to keep my voice."

Melle, a Ph.D. candidate and entrepreneur in New York City, with long, neat dreadlocks and a friendly manner, coparented for a couple of years with the father of her first child but has had two other children as a single mom. She's unusual in that she not only loves being a single mother, she thinks it's preferable. "For me," she says, "raising children and being with a man have to be two separate things. Marriage really does not create the best environment for child rearing." Melle's Ph.D. is in cultural history, and so she frames her opinion within the context of the cultural shift in the idea of marriage. Once upon a time, marriage was more of an economically necessary partnership. But as some of those economic and social pressures have been removed, the idea of marriage has become more romantic, sometimes unrealistically so. Nowadays, when shopping for a spouse, men and women both are looking for a soul mate, fantastic sex, and someone who will "get" them and tend to every last one of their emotional needs. That model, unstable on its own, falls apart completely when you add kids to the mix, Melle believes. So for her, single motherhood is, by definition, much better for the kids because they are the number one priority, and they aren't exposed to the conflict that so often arises in modern marriages when romantic expectations clash with child-rearing realities.

"When you're married, you're taking care of each other's adult needs, but it can be almost childish the way you want your needs met," Melle declares. That's fine when there aren't kids involved, but when there are? "You really can't spend a whole heck of a lot of time taking care of someone who *can* take care of themselves," she says. Melle says she sees, amongst her friends and acquaintances, two types of marriages with kids: "Ones where they work really well as coparents but the relationship suffers, or ones where the relationship is great but the kids are being raised by someone else [like a nanny]."

Melle loves men, she says, and men (and her kids' biological fathers) are a "vital part" of her life and the life of her kids. But given the isolating and often conflict-ridden nuclear family model our society works within today, she says, "I just don't think they're [ideally] an everyday part of it. There is this real serious dissonance between child rearing and marriage in our current society."

Melle's take on it is not at all representative of the majority of single moms by choice. Most, including me, still subscribe to the idea that two-parent families can work well, and that what they can offer both the children and the adult partners is well worth the challenges. Even if that's a fantasy, it's one I am not willing to give up.

I also like to believe that dads can be just as effective and involved parents as moms. As much as men are (rightly) criticized for often not stepping up to the parenting plate, they are also often (wrongly) shut out of parenting by a culture that positions the mom as the main hands-on parent. Even *Parenting* magazine has a tag line—"what matters to moms"—that tells dads that whatever's inside, it's not for them. Some men out there *are* taking paternity leave, making healthy dinners and careful decisions about laundry detergent, accompanying their toddlers to music class, selecting the right preschool, and changing diapers—but in doing so, they're having to risk being perceived as strange or unmanly. I think that's bad for everyone. At the same time, I can look around at married women talking about how their supposedly progressive husbands suddenly reverted to 1950s-style uninvolved dads when the kids came, and I can see, at least intellectually, that Melle may have a point.

## SERIAL MONOGAMY BUT NO KIDS

Whether they're too picky, too independent, or just unlucky in love, some single moms by choice just never could settle down.

"I've been a chronic dater," says Jamie, the children's book buyer who's now trying to conceive. "I'm a one-two-three date wonder, filling my friends' ears with stories."

"Every time I was at a party I would go home with somebody or end up with someone's phone number," echoes Kimberley, now the single mother of two. She was hardly at a loss for male companionship, but the relationships never got too serious. "I didn't have kids on my own because no one *picked* me—I haven't gotten married because I haven't found the person I want to be married to." Besides, she says, "I am a magnet for alcoholic crazy lunatics. I consider myself smart for not having married any of them!"

Other single moms did settle down, sometimes for many years, but didn't have kids right away and, then, like so many other women in these 50-percent-divorce-rate days, found themselves single again. Like me.

While I am not above having a one-night stand, I'm definitely the marrying kind. I love being tied down, being responsible to another person, sharing a home and a life. I had three long-term relationships during my prime baby-making years, and I dreamed of having kids with all of those partners. Partner one and I took concrete steps toward parenthood, but she wasn't ready to take the final plunge, and after eight years she decided she'd rather be single. Partner two and I actually bought a house in the suburbs with plenty of room for the kids, but after three years our relationship ended.

When I got together with partner three I was already thirty-eight and actively considering single motherhood. In fact, I remember shedding some tears, sharing with her my grief and fear about having to consider single motherhood . . . *while we were in the process of getting more deeply involved romantically!* Worse, she wanted children, too, and would have made a terrific mom. In one of my favorite pictures, she's lying in bed at my mom's house with my niece and nephew climbing all over her like little monkeys, having raced upstairs to wake her up because they were so excited to see her again. In my defense, our relationship was new (i.e., too soon to talk about kids) and my eggs were old (i.e., must have kids ASAP), and I saw the two issues as almost completely separate. Still, it's a wonder that she didn't dump me right there and then.

We were together, on and off, for three years, and part of what kept us together for so long was how much we both wanted kids and how well suited we were as potential coparents. But at last, we regretfully decided that we weren't the right match in other equally crucial ways. My first insemination happened to fall in the month we separated, and my excitement and hope for the future child were tempered by my sadness at leaving behind someone who in many ways was the perfect spouse, and who would have been a very loving parent to what I had spent a lot of time hoping would be our child.

Meanwhile, like several other women I spoke to, Michele, who works at a small family-run computer company in Toronto, was comfortably settled into the idea that she *did* have the perfect spouse. Or at least a serviceable one. "I was married for ten and a half years, and you always kind of think, oh, there's plenty of time to have kids," she says. After the divorce, "it hit me like a ton of bricks. I'm thirty-four years old and you're telling me if I want to have kids I have to start from *scratch*?!" Michele realized that that wasn't practical. At her age, to get fully established in another serious relationship could take forever, she thought. "If I want to do this before I'm too old, I better do it alone." So at age thirty-six, Michele is trying to get pregnant using anonymous donor sperm.

Debrah got married very young. "After a few years, he started talking about children, and I couldn't fathom having children with this man. I'm a very passionate person, and there wasn't much passion in the relationship." They divorced when she was twenty-six. Then she was in a relationship with a man she did want to have kids with. But Debrah, who originally had thought she wanted to go into family practice, decided to become a surgeon. Her boyfriend was a surgeon, and told her that he could not handle a two-surgeon relationship. "He always thought that his career would be the important one," Debrah says. She became a surgeon anyway, and the relationship ended. So for Debrah, deciding to become a single mom "wasn't the first time in my life I made a decision knowing it might have repercussions on my chances for a relationship in the future."

When Lisa M., a computer consultant in Concord, California, started trying to get pregnant, she was in a relationship with a woman who had two kids herself from a previous marriage. That relationship fell apart, partly because Lisa's partner didn't really want another kid. Despite being suddenly single, Lisa kept trying to conceive. "I knew I was ready to have a child," she says. "I was twenty-six, I had a good job, I had done all my ripping and running, my club-hopping and all that stuff. It was time. I couldn't put it on hold."

# "OOPS, I'M PREGNANT!" "ACCIDENTAL" PREGNANCY AS CATALYST

Other than birthdays, breakups, and dating insanity, "accidental" pregnancies seem to be the most common way of sliding into single motherhood, making what is really a choice seem like more of a happy mishap. When I was in my late thirties and between relationships with women, I dated a couple of guys, and I'll admit that, as wrongheaded as I believe it to be, I was tempted to chance such an "accident" myself. In fact, I told friends at the time, I felt like I should have had a giant neon sign on my forehead: WARNING! I WILL TRICK YOU INTO GETTING ME PREGNANT! I didn't do it (after twenty years in the gay community and a job at an HIV magazine, I am exceptionally well versed in the reasons for practicing safer sex, never mind the questionable morality of using a date as a donor), but, boy, was it on my mind. An "oops!" pregnancy would have presented its own challenges, to be sure, emotionally, legally, and STD-wise, but in other ways it would have been so much easier (and cheaper and more fun) than becoming a single mom the dull, premeditated, clinical way that I did. If the women I've talked to are any indication, the midthirties are rife with such "accidents." For a couple of these women, the "accident" ended in miscarriage, but the experience showed them that single motherhood wasn't as scary as they might have thought, and they decided to pursue it more openly.

After her divorce, freaking out about how she was going to have kids as a suddenly single thirty-four-year-old, Michele had an "accidental" pregnancy. She was "terrified" at what people would think, she says. Nevertheless, she decided to keep the child—but not the boyfriend. "This was not by any means a serious relationship," Michele explains. "I told him I didn't want involvement and he was fine with that." What Michele didn't expect was the overwhelmingly positive reaction she got from her family and friends. "They were just ecstatic for me," she says. "I was so blown away at how supportive everyone was." It turns out that they all knew how much she wanted kids, and after her divorce their biggest concern was that she wouldn't have the chance to be a mom.

Michele's accidental pregnancy ended in miscarriage, but the experience gave her the courage to seek out pregnancy in a more thought-out way. "There's not a stigma anymore," she says.

Laura, a photo editor in New York, says, "back when I was thirty-six I thought I had until I was forty to get pregnant." So when she was forty and dating someone she thought she was going to marry, "I pretty much just stopped using birth control." At forty-one, she got pregnant by her would-be fiancé. It did not turn out the way she had hoped. He split. And then she miscarried. "After that, I gave up on a lot of things," Laura recalls. But as her forties marched on, she still skipped birth control—and held out a glimmer of hope. Sure enough, at forty-three, Laura was pregnant again. Her then-boyfriend was horrified: "He broke up with me immediately." Three months later, she miscarried again. But having stayed pregnant longer "sort of ignited my hope," Laura says. "Maybe I still had what it takes to produce a child—and forget the man."

Sometimes an accidental pregnancy really is an accident. "I didn't exactly choose it from the beginning," admits Erron, a twenty-eight-year-old ob-gyn resident at Dartmouth Medical School in New Hampshire, who now identifies as a single mother by choice. She'd been in a relationship for six years and was on the Pill. Which failed. Her boyfriend wanted her to get an abortion. Erron considered it—certainly heading into eighty-hour weeks as a resident was a terrible time to have a baby—but says, "to be honest with you, I was doing a rotation on family planning. Just seeing the abortions, I couldn't choose it for myself." Besides, she reasoned, there would never be a good time. The accidental pregnancy forced Erron to sit down and do the mental math. If she waited to have kids until she was through with all her training, she'd be thirty-five—at the end of the peak fertility years, still possibly without a relationship, plus older and probably more burned out. As crazy as it might have seemed to her before the positive pregnancy test, she realized now was as good a time as any.

At thirty-eight, Amy, a Washington, D.C., economist, is ready to become a single mom on purpose through anonymous donor insemination. The story of how she got to that point—through an accidental first pregnancy—is just about the worst one I have heard. For several years, Amy had been "nesting and socking away money." Looking back on it, she realizes she was at cross-purposes. "There were actions and behaviors of mine that suggested I was preparing myself for single motherhood, but I was nowhere near ready to order up donor sperm and do it like that." Then, at thirty-seven, Amy got pregnant "accidentally."

"I never would have used deceit, but, yeah, it was kind of by accident and kind of not," she admits. "After a month of unprotected sex, I thought, well, that's a terrible approach. But I was already pregnant."

It turned out that Amy's "casual" boyfriend didn't feel so casual about her and wanted kids, so when she didn't want to marry him, he became very angry. Her pregnancy was physically miserable and emotionally isolating, with no support system in place. She had an unsympathetic mother, her obstetrical practice seemed disapproving of her single-mom status—and there was evidence that the fetus might have birth defects. Despite all that, Amy gave birth to a perfect baby boy—and was slammed with severe postpartum depression. Then, at eleven weeks, just as she was starting therapy for her depression and things were looking up, her healthy little boy, "the chubbiest, roundest thing," died of sudden infant death syndrome.

"I did not want to live," Amy says of the period after her son's death. "And if not for the gift of a therapist I had a connection with, I would not have made it."

She also reached out and found the group Single Mothers by Choice. "I went to a workshop and realized that there were a lot of other women like me, and if I did it [got pregnant] again I would have a whole community behind me. There's a way to do it without having a partner that you're not in love with and not on the same page with."

Though she is still grieving and trying to heal, Amy feels like she has learned so much from the other single moms about resources and networking and building a support system. Because of that, she can see that a purposeful pregnancy as a single mother would be a totally different experience from her difficult first one—and she knows that the tragedy of SIDS is unlikely to happen twice. "I was really leery of the sperm-donor route before," Amy says. "I wouldn't have done it. I was worried about what other people might think. I thought there was a big stigma." But her accidental pregnancy, though not strictly accidental, turned that around. With the exception of her mother, she says, "people were so supportive. People were so happy for me that I thought maybe I could do this on my own."

## SOUNDING THE BIOLOGICAL
## FIRE ALARM

Most biological clocks just tick with increasing volume. But for a few unlucky women, they are wired like bombs. Nina, the project manager
from Baltimore, had a head-on collision with her biological clock—in her
doctor's office. Nina had a "borderline cancerous" tumor removed from her
uterus at age twenty-five, and her doctor told her that if she wanted kids she
should have them ASAP: "You should definitely do it before you're thirty,
because we need to take everything out." When Nina hit thirty, she told the
doc, "Well, I'm not ready. Can I have an extension?" After several such "ex-
tensions," her doctor told her she couldn't have any more. "At thirty-six, you
have to have a hysterectomy," he said. "It's kind of weird having your doctor push the alarm button on your biological clock," Nina notes. But, pushed
against the wall, the decision was clear for her. "I've always loved children.
In college during the summer I would nanny, and my degree is in theater for
young audiences," she says. "I thought, I don't want to be a single mom, but
I don't want to be fifty and look back and say, 'You know what, I really wish
I had children.' "

A similar thing happened to Jocelyn, a psychologist from Arizona who is
now the single mom of a fifteen-year-old. Only Jocelyn did not get an early
heads-up. After a "difficult marriage," she got divorced at thirty-seven. At
her next checkup, she asked her doctor how much time she had to have kids.
"You don't have any time," she replied flatly. A visit to a fertility specialist
confirmed it. "The reproductive endocrinologist told me I was going into
menopause. I really didn't have time to piddle around and contemplate my
navel." It was a shock. "It was a dark time," Jocelyn admits. This was around
1991—there weren't any books to read or groups to join. "I was trying to sort
through the fear," she says. "I had to make the choice in a vacuum." Jocelyn
decided to try to get pregnant on her own, and quickly, through donor insemination. "Even though I was terrified and feeling very alone, I knew if I
didn't do it I'd be such an angry and bitter person for the rest of my life."
Luckily, she was able to conceive. But there are many women who have
similar stories—without the happy ending.

## SINGLE MOMS WHO AREN'T SINGLE

When you separate love and marriage from the baby carriage, sometimes it turns out you can have all of it, after all. I talked to a number of women who are single in parenthood and who live alone, but who are coupled in love. I'm way too clingy to imagine this working for me—if I love someone I want them next to me every night. Even though I'm extremely tall, I find a king-size bed to be a cold, vast expanse of tundra, too big for two people. I threw a fit once when my partner told an airline agent that it was just fine if we sat several rows apart during a transcontinental flight—she didn't even *try* to get us seated together. (I get mad all over again just thinking about it!) Basically, I have the personal-space requirements of your average golden retriever. And I can't imagine having a partner who wasn't also a coparent. But retaining larger than average amounts of independence works beautifully for some couples.

In fact, Mikki Morrissette, the author of *Choosing Single Motherhood: The Thinking Woman's Guide* and the leader of a single motherhood movement of sorts, is actually happily married—to a man who lives thirty minutes away from her home in Minneapolis. They fell in love when she was five months pregnant with her second child, whom she had conceived as a single mom. As a parent, she's still single. Her husband was a widower raising two older kids alone, one of them an emotionally volatile, sometimes aggressive special-needs child. Merging their households, with Mikki's two young children, would not have been a good thing for any of the kids, they felt. So instead of cohabitating and coparenting, they get together for "date night" once a week—for both of them, a much-needed break from single parenting—see each other on some weekends and special occasions, and talk on the phone a lot. "It took a lot of adjustments on both sides to make such an unusual marriage work," she says, but it really does. "Seeing each other so seldom really keeps it fresh," Mikki says. "We don't have the minutiae of everyday life."

Miriam, an accountant, has been with her current boyfriend for two and a half years. She lives in a town house in Philadelphia with her Yorkie, and he lives in the mountains an hour and a half away. They see each other every weekend, sometimes during the week as well, and they talk and e-mail daily.

With her career in accounting still in its growth phase, she has no plans to move to the country anytime soon, and he's allergic to the city. But it works. "We're both independent people and we're both not needy or codependent," she says. "I don't think I've ever been this happy," she declares. "He's exactly what I always wanted in a man, and the relationship is exactly what I wanted." Except: She wants kids, and her boyfriend doesn't want more—he has three from his previous marriage.

"Are you sure you don't want more children?" she recently asked him.

"Yes, I'm sure."

It wasn't a financial issue, Miriam says. He has three kids he doesn't see every day, and he feels guilty about that. With her, "he'd be biologically creating another child who he wouldn't see every day. He'd want to be in birthing classes with me and in the delivery room, and he can't promise that." For him, the moral decision was to say yes to Miriam, but no to fatherhood.

"Well, do you mind if I try?" Miriam asked.

He didn't mind.

"You know people are going to assume it's your child anyway," Miriam told him.

"I don't have a problem with that," was his reply.

So she's trying, setting out on a very unfamiliar road to family, but hopeful and happy.

## GETTING PAST THE FREAK FACTOR

When you go bungee-jumping, skydiving, jumping off a cliff, all those leap-of-faith-type activities, you kind of want someone else to go before you, right? So it is with choosing to be a single mom—especially for women who come from communities where having a baby without a father or wedding ring is uncommon or nonexistent. Women want answers to three main questions: Can it really be done? Do the kids turn out OK? And, perhaps most important, If I do this, will I be a total freak? Meeting others who have done it can provide some answers.

A few years ago, through mutual friends, Kimberley ended up at a barbecue with actress Jodie Foster. The talk turned to Kimberley's desire for kids, and Jodie, who has two sons with no father in the picture, said, "You know, you don't have to get married to have a baby." But to Kimberley, that seemed about as realistic as any other aspect of Hollywood stardom. "In my mind, only celebrities could do that," says Kimberley. It wasn't until another friend of a friend became a single mother that the idea started to take hold. "*She* can do that?" Kimberley remembers exclaiming. Here was someone who was very much a regular person, and she was doing just fine as a single mom. "If she can do that, *I* can do that!" Just a few years later, Kimberley was the happy single mother of two.

"I'd had the idea in the back of my mind for a long time," says Samantha, who works for a trade association in Washington, D.C. "I think I'd read an article about it in college." As she inched past thirty, she joined the national group Single Mothers by Choice, but in a passive way, just getting the quarterly newsletter. Meanwhile, like a kid who wants her friend to be the first one to try something scary, she was active in encouraging an older friend to go the single motherhood route. "I wanted her to be my role model," Samantha admits.

When she turned thirty-six and was "seeing another commitmentphobe," Samantha finally took a bigger step.

"One day I was PMSing and I got out all the old newsletters, joined the Listserv, joined the local group, and went to their picnic that weekend," she says.

Talking to other women made all the difference. "I thought, these are really cool, attractive, normal women," Samantha says, not the "ugly losers" she'd feared they might be. "They'd just had bad luck with men, like me. It made it seem like more of a normal thing to do." Also, she met older women in the group who had waited until they were forty and had experienced expensive and heartbreaking fertility challenges. They warned her against making the same mistake. "People said, if you're really serious about this, don't wait." Samantha called and made the doctor's appointment that week. "I actually gave my boyfriend a chance to stop me," she says. "But he wasn't willing to make the relationship less casual." About six months later, she was pregnant from an anonymous donor. And now her older friend has a child as a single mom, too—with Samantha as her role model.

For Miriam, it was also a Single Mothers by Choice event—a barbecue—that "cemented my decision to go through with this," she says. "Seeing all these happy moms and happy kids really made me excited and know that this was what I wanted to do." One woman in particular inspired her—she'd just had twins through in vitro fertilization. "She had hired help but no support system at all—and she was pretty happy," Miriam remembers. "I thought, if she can do it with her limited support system, then I can certainly do it with my support system."

Role models made the difference for Nicole, too. She'd gone so far as to look at online sperm banks, but "they served couples," she says, and thought, I don't want to be a footnote. At a barbecue, she happened to meet a woman who'd conceived at a clinic, with an anonymous sperm donor. "That was the key to everything," she says. Through that woman, she met other single moms by choice, "and their kids, which was key," Nicole says. "I know this sounds silly, but emotionally I needed to see that their kids were the same as other kids."

As part of her research, Debrah went on a Single Mothers by Choice vacation in Colorado. "I wanted to see how some of these women were dealing with things—what they found helpful, what they found difficult." It was a useful fact-finding trip. "Each had her own way of doing things," Debrah remembers, "but they all made it work." The result for Debrah? "It became less of an off-the-wall thing to do or think about."

Sometimes if you don't have a role model or a support group, the best thing to do is to create one yourself. That's what my friend Julie did. In her late thirties, Julie was a lesbian wannabe-mom who still hadn't found a life partner. She didn't want to be a single mom, but the clock was ticking. Instead of giving in to the angst and isolation, she created her own community by starting a support group for single lesbian moms and wannabe moms. It helped her through the decision and her pregnancy, and though the group eventually disbanded, "I'm still friends with some of those people," Julie says.

For most of the middle-class white women I spoke to, having a baby solo, whether by choice or by accident, was virtually unheard of in their communities, so getting support has been crucial. But most of the (also middle-class) Black women I interviewed had the opposite challenge. Single motherhood may not have been what they expected for themselves or what their parents wanted for them, but it was far from unheard of in the Black community. For them, choosing to be a single mom meant embracing or allowing themselves to be seen as what was for some of them an uncomfortable stereotype: the ubiquitous single Black mother. Alice, who is Black, is a West Point graduate and business executive who pulls in a huge salary. "I don't want to be thought of as a stereotypical careless single mother," she says—but because of her race it happens. "I just had to get over it."

## PARENTS AS PUSHERS: "WE WANT GRANDKIDS AND WE DON'T REALLY CARE HOW YOU GET 'EM"

For many women, the scariest part of considering single motherhood is, "What will my parents think?" For the majority of women I spoke to, this fear turns out to be totally unnecessary. Most are surprised to find their families more receptive to it than they'd expected. I was surprised, too. Honestly, as a New York City resident, I assumed I was cozily cocooned in a liberal fantasyland rivaled only by San Francisco, and that in other, more normal parts of the country, the experience of choosing single motherhood would be marked by a fair amount of stigma and strife. Not so. Turns out, Toto, that times have really changed: even Kansas isn't in Kansas anymore. And for more women than I'd ever have guessed, the prospective grandparents were the ones to float the idea of single motherhood.

Alice, a telecommunications executive in Maryland, was single and approaching her fortieth birthday when her mom said, "I think you should be a mother."

"Explain that to me; how would that work?" Alice, a former captain in the army, remembers saying.

"Well, I'll help," said her mother, who Alice describes as "a very conservative, very traditional" woman who has been married forty-five years.

"I had never thought to get pregnant without getting married," Alice says. "I'm a fairly progressive person, and it was a shock to me that she had gotten to a place that I hadn't gotten to."

Debrah, the surgeon who was married once and has had several long-term relationships, says that, when she was in her late thirties and single, she was talking with her mom about marriage and kids. "Maybe you'll have to think about things separately," her mother suggested.

"I've always had boyfriends," declares Miriam. "There was a time in my mid- to late twenties when I was in a lot of relationships, but they weren't working out." Miriam's mom was in the medical profession and suggested she consider single motherhood through an anonymous sperm donor. "I might've been thinking about it in an abstract form, but my mom was the one who made it tangible."

When Diana, a university professor from Des Moines, was thirty-four, she told her mother, a social worker, that she wanted to start thinking about whether or not to have a child someday. "That conversation got the ball rolling. My parents were eager to have a grandchild and started brainstorming with me," Diana says. "It was actually my dad who suggested I use an anonymous donor. He's a doctor, and had friends from med school who had been sperm donors." Over the course of the ongoing conversation with her parents and her sister, the idea of becoming a single parent by choice came to seem more and more normal and attractive to Diana: "They all promised and reassured me that I would not be in this alone, that my having a child would be a family project, and that they would be involved and help in whatever ways they could, even though they lived far away." Even with family support, "it was an act of faith. I was terrified about how my life would change," she said. "But I thought if I don't do it, I might regret it." And her sister, an obstetrician who knew the risks of waiting to conceive, said, "If you think you might do this at thirty-seven, just do it now." She realized her sister was right. "I can always have a relationship, but I can't always have a baby." Besides, the timing was getting too tight. "If I started a relationship, it would be at least a year or two before I was sure enough to have kids with that person."

Lisa S., an elementary schoolteacher from Milwaukee, was married in her twenties. By the time she was thirty-five she had a ten-year-old daughter and had long been divorced. "Since my marriage, I'd been through two very serious relationships," says Lisa, a redhead with lively blue eyes—but neither worked out. She started thinking about a second child on her own. Finally, she confided in her mother. "My mother looked at me and said, 'What took you so long? Having a kid is the one thing that gives you more joy than anything else. Your dad and I actually talked about it and wondered whether you might do it.'"

## THE PLUSES OF PARENTING SOLO

Single motherhood is far from most women's first choice, and the commonly held assumption is that it only offers negatives when held up against parenting with a partner. Indeed, it was Plan B for the vast majority of the women I spoke to. But this is a glass-half-full bunch, and so many of the single moms I spoke to talked about unexpected ways that single motherhood is better, and easier. You've got total responsibility, to be sure, but you've also got total control and freedom.

I got a tiny taste of what that means just the other night, when I had a couple over for dinner. They brought their eighteen-month-old daughter, who they put to bed in my son Scott's Pack 'N Play. When it was time to go, it was snowing, and they started bickering about the right way to get the sleeping baby home. "Let's just put her in the stroller and cover her with blankets so we don't wake her up," one of them said. "She'll be warm enough."

"No, we have to put her coat on!" said the other one in a way that did not invite debate.

"This is the downside of having two parents," the first one mumbled as she headed down the hall obediently, tiny coat in hand.

"There's a lot of things I prefer about the idea of doing it alone," says Michele. For one thing, she says, in this age of divorce, you'll never have to explain to your child "why Daddy's no longer here."

For straight women, it's also a free ticket out of the sex wars. "My ex-husband would still be playing as much golf as ever," Michele declares. "He wouldn't change his lifestyle to fit the circumstances. I've watched so many couples where they're equal partners until the child comes along, and then suddenly it's 'You're the mother, you stay home.' I also know a family where the son always goes hunting and fishing with his dad, but the daughter is never invited. Those gender differences drive me crazy, and this way I don't have to deal with them."

"I won't get any help, but I won't be disappointed by anyone, either," Michele says—something that's true for single moms of any sexual orientation. "There's no arguing over 'I got up last time to change the diaper.'"

Ellen, the single mother of two, agrees. "I don't have this aggravation of expecting something from someone," she says. "It's exhausting enough taking care of two kids without being pissed off at someone for failing you." Ellen's boss, who is married, told her that he developed an appreciation for the benefits of single parenthood after his wife left town for a week, leaving him in sole charge of their two boys. "He said it was easier knowing it was all up to you, rather than thinking you had a partner and being like, 'What have *you* done recently? *I've* done this, this, and this.'"

The benefits don't end there. "I'm so grateful that no matter what happens in life, I will never have to fight for custody of my kids," Ellen says. "My married friends can't say that."

Jocelyn, the psychologist from Phoenix, was married during her prime babymaking years. But she and her husband never had kids because "he wasn't ready—he was always trying to get himself established and stabilized." After they divorced when Jocelyn was thirty-eight, he remarried and almost immediately had a kid—then divorced his second wife when the kid was about two and a half. *Not* having kids within her marriage to him, Jocelyn concludes, "was the best dumb luck I ever had." Her kid hasn't had to deal with the instability and negativity of divorce. And doing it alone, for Jocelyn, has been a joy and a revelation. "I didn't come from the Cleavers," she says, and she thought it was near impossible to raise children without screwing them up. Raising her daughter, who is now fifteen, has been "extremely healing," she says, and the control she's had as a single parent has helped. "I have found that if you really work hard, if you do read all the books, your child will turn out OK."

Diana, now the single mother of two, thinks single motherhood is beneficial for both her daughter and son because "I can give my children a model of a strong, capable woman." She says also that people feel freer to help out a single mom: "They feel like they have a place." And she thinks single motherhood by choice can create an optimal situation for finding a partner, which she recently has—she's about to marry her boyfriend of almost four years. "You can wait for the right person and relationship. You don't end up marrying somebody just because you're anxious to have kids."

Two of the moms I spoke to have done it both ways—with the dad and without one—and for one of them, single motherhood comes out ahead. "I can tell you how hard it is to be a single mom," says Anne. "There's nobody to pick up the slack for you. There *is* no slack." Still, she says, "I don't think I would trade it for the other."

When Anne was thirty-four, she and her boyfriend had an unplanned pregnancy, and decided to keep the kid. "We stayed together for two years afterward, but certainly having the kid contributed to the split-up."

When Anne's daughter was five, Anne decided to have another child, this time as a single mom by choice. "I'm the kind of person who's like, 'I can do this, I'm a strong person.' " Her friends and family thought she was nuts. But, Anne says, she had an advantage other women don't when contemplating single motherhood: "I knew what it felt like to be completely in love with a child. If you don't have a child, you have to just trust it will all be worth it. So for me, it wasn't so great of a leap."

It's been totally worth it, she says, and she finds that total responsibility isn't a burden, it's freedom: "I have one kid who's all mine and nobody can ever fuck with that," she says, "and another kid who I always have to do this dance of how she's to be raised." Anne also thinks single motherhood can be better for the kids. "Single moms' kids are more socially well adjusted," she believes, "because you have to rely on others. You have to get your family involved; you have to get babysitters. These kids are used to being part of a wider community." Anne also feels that single moms' kids don't become the overindulged monsters that some partnered parents turn out. As a single mom, Anne says, "you don't have time to sit and negotiate with a child who's upset that the bread isn't buttered all the way to the edge."

Most of all, she says, a single mom has the clarity of knowing she has to do everything, instead of being in a position to rely on a partner who might let her down. "There are very few straight couples I know where the men really pull their weight," Anne says. Her relationship was no exception. "After my breakup, I was still doing all the child care. The difference is, I was now doing it without all this bitterness that was driving me crazy."

## THERE'S SUCH A THING AS TOO MANY DUCKS: PREPARATION VERSUS PROCRASTINATION

Before becoming a single mom, it's important to put your ducks in a row. Financial ducks, emotional ducks, practical ducks. Like many of the women I spoke to, I moved to a bigger apartment in a family neighborhood. I made sure I had a decent financial cushion. I tried to do as much angsting as possible before the baby came, so as to avoid freaking out afterward. "I even went to see a social worker for three or four sessions," says Marcy. "I wanted to do the right thing for the right reasons." But if you focus too much on lining up ducks, you may end up waiting until it's too late for motherhood. "After a while, I stopped all the research," Nicole remembers. "There's such a thing as too much information."

Elisa, an independent sales representative based in San Francisco, was forty-one when she realized she really wanted a child—but she would have preferred to wait another ten years: "I lived in a small apartment, I didn't think I could afford it." But what with being female and wanting to have a biological child, she realized her choices boiled down to having a baby now or never. "I could not read another article about a woman in her late thirties who found she couldn't have children. I would get physically ill." So despite normally being a "logistical queen," Elisa didn't think much further than that bottom line. There have been major struggles in the two years since she's had her daughter, but Elisa says she's so happy to be a mom and glad she didn't look too much before she leaped: "If I had looked at can I afford it, do I have room for it, I never would have done it."

One woman I know actually became the coordinator of a wannabe-single-mom's support group when she was thirty-eight. Five years later, most of the women in the group have kids, and she is still childless, trying to get everything in perfect shape, trying to make it all neat and logical and rational and safe. But like love, like sex, like life itself, becoming a parent isn't any of those things. Having a kid, especially as a single mom, is like jumping off a cliff. At a certain point you've just got to hold your breath and do it.

The ticktock of that bio-clock is what drives most of us to take the leap. One single mother told me: "You never wake up and say, I'm ready. I'm ready to give up my night's sleep, I'm ready to give up my privacy in the bathroom, all my free time. . . . It's just never going to happen!" Single moms will tell you it's the best thing they've ever done—and many will also tell you they wish they'd done it earlier.

"The thing I would most like to tell thinkers," says Samantha, "is that it's not as hard as you think it will be, and you don't have to figure out every detail in advance. When my daughter was born a year ago, I lived in a one-bedroom apartment and had no local family, and it's all worked out fine."

"I was so late in getting to this because I resisted so long having a baby without a partner," says Laura, who eventually had twins at age forty-four, using donor egg and donor sperm. "I squandered eight years. I really wish I had made the decision earlier. Every time I hear a thirty-six-year-old say she's going to put it off for a year, I cringe.

"It's not just me that's old," Laura adds. "My mother's seventy-nine," she says, and not physically in good enough shape to play with her grandsons or babysit them, and not likely to be around long in their lives. "That's heart-breaking."

There are many women who wait so long that biological parenthood is no longer an option, and still-single motherhood can seem too scary a path to take. Of the women I spoke to, Frances, a slender fitness instructor in New York City with chin-length black hair and a smooth, pretty face, wins the procrastination prize. Frances started trying to get pregnant when she was forty and married. Her attempts at pregnancy failed and soon enough she was divorced anyway, wondering, "What was I thinking when I married *him?*" She tried conceiving again, with the help of fertility drugs, when she was in another relationship at forty-five, but it wasn't working and the drugs were wreaking havoc on her body: "My right ovary kept on getting bigger and bigger and bigger," she says. Besides, "the whole fertility process put a strain on the relationship." Which eventually ended. She didn't want to do more medical intervention—"I probably would have had to do donor egg and donor sperm, and that was too weird for me," Frances recalls, in her low, husky voice with its hint of a New York accent. "I decided it was better to adopt somebody who needed a home." But she still couldn't imagine being a single mom. She was in a service industry—how could she afford it? Still, "I didn't want to leave this planet without somebody calling me Mom." Year after year, she vowed to do it—"next year." Finally her sister said, "Every year you have a different excuse. This is going to pass you by. You're so full of shit. Go get a colonic!" At fifty-three—the last year any adoption agency would let her adopt—Frances adopted an infant girl from Guatemala. "It wasn't a good time for me, but my back was against the wall," she remembers.

"It's the best thing I ever did in my life," Frances asserts, becoming so emotional that she starts to cry. "I never knew that I could love somebody this way, ever. There isn't anything in my life that is better than this."

That said, though, she paid a price for waiting. She'd wanted a biological child—yet it had apparently been too late for that at forty, and then she went through expensive and unsuccessful fertility treatments. And now, as young as she appears and as happy as she is with her decision, she is the fifty-eight-year-old mother of a four-year-old.

"I'm an oddity," Frances admits. "You don't find many women at my age who have a small child. And what I've found in the dating situation is the people I go out with usually have grown children, so they're not interested in dating somebody with a small child." Her current boyfriend has a preteen and a young teen, "so they're not too far removed," she says.

"I had all these fears," Frances concludes, "and I let my fears stop me from doing it earlier. This is the best thing I've ever done, but I wish I had done it earlier." Her advice to other women? "Do it. Somehow the universe provides."

# Buying Dad

## *How to Make the Most Natural Thing in the World Unnatural*

J enny, who is straight, was working with a group of kids when one of the kids' lesbian moms noticed her affinity for children.

"Do you want kids?" the mom asked.

"Yeah," said Jenny.

"Are you with someone?"

"No," Jenny said.

"Well, all you need is a credit card," the mom replied.

"I'd never thought of it," Jenny said. "I'm straight and I thought I'd find a man, get married to a man, have sex with the man, and then have a baby with the man." But as she approached her midthirties, the credit-card approach started to make a lot of sense.

The lesbian mom was being glib, but indeed, as wannabe single mothers, many of us find ourselves practically signing over our paychecks to the infertility industry—when often the only reason we're "infertile" is because we don't have a man. In addition to doctor's fees, we pay up to five hundred dollars a vial for a tiny amount of semen from some guy we've never laid eyes on—who our kid may end up looking and acting like. "Doesn't that all seem a little dehumanizing?" someone once asked me. Uh, *yeah*. And a little crazy to be paying for something so widely available for free. After throwing a couple of thousand bucks into artificial insemination, even the most hard-core lesbians start to notice that cute waiter at the corner bistro—never mind how crazy buying sperm can seem if you're straight. Yet the sperm-bank route is often the best and most responsible choice for those who can afford it. You're not risking your health and safety with a one-night stand, you're not tricking anyone into fatherhood, and you're not entering into a lifelong and potentially conflict-ridden legal and emotional relationship with someone you intend to be a father but not a parent.

Still, it can be hard to wrap your head around. "My best friend's mom is the most straitlaced, churchgoing woman you've ever met," says Nicole, who is trying to conceive using anonymous donor sperm. "And she said, 'Why don't you just go to a bar?'" But Nicole doesn't feel that's a viable option. "It's just too fraught with danger"—of violence, or of contracting HIV or other sexually transmitted diseases. Besides, she says, "if the guy didn't know about it, it just isn't right, and it wouldn't be fair to him."

So how does it work to buy Dad? There are dozens of sperm banks all across the country, and most have Web sites. As a result, searching for a donor is like online dating meets online shopping meets tenth-grade biology (remember Mendel's hybrid pea plants?) meets the American Kennel Club. Weird doesn't even begin to describe it.

"It was so bizarre going on the Internet, picking out the father of your child like you're picking out shoes," says Miriam. "I felt like Madeline Kahn as Empress Nympho, picking escorts," she says, referring to the Mel Brooks comedy *History of the World*: "Yes, no, no, no, no, yes."

Indeed, on many sites, you can shop for your favorite donor eye color from the same kind of drop-down menu other e-commerce sites use to distinguish the navy kitten-heel mules from the same model in red or brown. Even though single women and lesbian couples now make up nearly half their customers, the banks are still set up with the focus on hair color, eye color, skin color, and height—the original idea being to physically approximate the customer's infertile husband. Most banks tend to spend little time on the more complex (and subjective) qualities, like personality, that are of interest to many single or lesbian women, who often don't have one particular physical description in mind. So when you're looking for a donor, you often have to come up with what is essentially a racial profile before the sperm bank's database will furnish any other information.

The next step is to browse through "short profiles" of donors, a service that is free of charge. These paragraph-long (or shorter) profiles have a general description of the man—who is assigned a number—with his profession or college major and a summary of his family health history. If one interests you, you just type in your credit card number and you can order more "products." The basic package (fifteen dollars and up for each donor) includes a questionnaire the donor filled out, his health history, and a health history of his extended family. Then some banks also offer more information if you want to pay extra for it. These additional products (costing about ten to twenty-five dollars apiece) can include an audio interview with the donor, his results on standard temperament tests, and baby pictures of him—in some cases you can even order an adult picture of the guy (though no picture at all is the industry norm). There are often different price categories of donors—a donor with a B.A. might be cheaper than a donor with a Ph.D., for example. And an open-identity donor—that's one who has agreed that any children resulting from his donation can contact him when they reach age eighteen—costs more than a donor who wants to remain anonymous forever. Once you've made your selection, you have to get your doctor to send in a form saying, basically, that you're in good breeding condition and you're all set to receive shipments of semen. If you've chosen a popular donor, however, you may have to wait for him. And there are limits (voluntarily set by each bank) on how many women can bear a child with one donor. At my bank, the limit was fifteen. So you may pick a donor and then have to stop using him once he's maxed out.

Needless to say, despite the pluses of anonymous donor insemination, some of us find it easier to swallow than others.

For Min, choosing a donor was "kind of excruciating. I did not have one pleasant experience, but I have a sense of humor about it." One bank was all business, she said, adopting an infomercial-sales-pitch voice: "and, for seven dollars more, you can have . . .' "

"I was turned off by that," Min says. "Then they told me if the guy was educated his sperm would cost more, and I found that shocking. Very often they would talk about the guy's nose, and I found that a little anti-Semitic." The whole process was weird and upsetting for Min. "Every little piece of information like that took me a little time to digest," she says.

Min decided she wanted an open donor with a good family health history and a proven track record of pregnancies. "Initially, it sort of freaked me out that the guy would have other children running around," she says, "but with each birthday I realized I had to get over that." As her own fertility be-came more doubtful with age, she felt, "I needed to go with someone who had a proven track record."

One of the donors she picked because "the man wrote something really beautiful," she says. Another made the cut because there seemed to be some uncanny overlaps: "He was an artist and a teacher, I'm an artist and a teacher. His mother was a speech pathologist, my mother is a speech pathologist." But ultimately, Min does not feel such things matter. "How picky can we get, you know?" she says. If the medical history is good, that should be good enough. And with time, the process seems less weird and the donor's particulars less important. "It's about the child," she says.

The experience of shopping for sperm does get a little easier the longer you're at it. But for some women, the process is fairly easy from the start. They feel that sperm is sperm is sperm, and as long as the donor is healthy, the rest is of little importance.

The particulars of the anonymous donor "didn't really matter to me," re-members Michele. She wanted someone tall and in good health, but other than that, it was all the same to her. "Friends I showed the list to were more interested in it than I was," she says. "It's gonna be *my* kid," she points out— "what do I care what the other person is like?" Besides, she says, even when you know the other person intimately, there are no guarantees about what the kids will be like. "I've known enough people where both parents are really tall and the kid is really short—you never know what's gonna happen."

"Education, signs of intelligent life were important to me," says Diana, who also didn't really sweat the decision. "In the end, the most important thing was medical health. I chose the sperm bank [I did] because they did more thorough health testing than some others."

"People seem very attached to their donors," Debrah observes, "but there was nothing emotional about it for me. I looked for physical characteristics that were very much like my own. I wanted some athletic ability, some music ability, and some academic ability. For me, it was a logical thing."

Liz had trouble with it at first—she spent a full year looking at donors. Finally, she decided it was ridiculous to focus on it too much: "I would never be this scrutinous of someone I was dating," she realized. She backed off. "I looked to make sure they weren't crazy," then focused on other basics, like looks compatible with hers and good health.

"You don't know anything about this guy, I guess that's true," says Jessica, a New York City small-business owner who has a daughter from anonymous-donor insemination. But she was not too uncomfortable with it, especially since her donor was given "every available blood test" and was interviewed extensively by the sperm bank. "What do you really know about half the people you date?"

## GUY OR GAMETE?

Women are divided on how much importance they place on donor selection, and whether they think of the donor as a person—the father of their child—or as a collection of chromosomes. How they think often has a lot to do with where they stand on the nature-nurture debate. Though, according to Wellesley sociologist Rosanna Hertz, author of *Single by Chance, Mothers by Choice*, some single moms of the "nurture" persuasion end up putting more stock in "nature" once they get to know their kids and see unexplained mannerisms and personality traits. A donor who was seen only as chromosomes can start to develop into more of a complete person in the mother's mind, Hertz says, once she sees the influence his personality seems to have on her child.

"Some people are so clinical about it," Jamie says. "They think of the donor as just sperm. But it is a person, and it is half of my child's DNA." So Jamie chose a donor who seemed to have a nice personality—"I really did what I've done with online dating, I went with my gut."

Shannon also saw the donor as a guy, not just a gamete, and that made her search more difficult. "I spent months poring over the Internet trying to find out about every single sperm bank in existence," she recalls. "I wrote out little comparison charts—height, weight, complexion, ethnicity, hair, eye color, health, personality, interests, schooling—and looked at who I thought would be the kind of man I would want to be the father of my child."

"As a conservative woman who only wants to consider conservative sperm, I find that there is a big choice for leftist sperm but not so much for more right-wing seed," says Jennifer, a wannabe single mom in Toronto who is only partly joking. For her it's about nature but also about normalizing the experience somewhat. "I want to believe that I'd like and respect the donor as a person, even if my future child or I were never to meet him. Genetic predisposition as related to politics aside, I need to believe that this is a guy with a good head on his shoulders who does not see this world in a completely different way than I do."

I probably would have been quite solidly on the nurture side of the debate, if it weren't for the somewhat unusual details of my family. When my dad married my mom, he already had four kids from a previous marriage. He died (heart attack, age forty-two) when I was twenty-two months old. Since our father was dead and my half siblings lived with their mom, I never really got to know them—socially, they were more like distant cousins to me. Then, sixteen years later, I visited my older half sister for a month and was amazed at the similarities in our personalities. We had a lot of the same character traits—good and bad. And people kept telling us we looked alike, which must have meant we have similar mannerisms since our features are different. Before getting to know Jane, I had always thought I was a lot like my mother. Instead, I realized that what my mom had always told me was true: in personality and temperament, I definitely took after my father's side of the family. And, though my brother gets a lot of his temperament from my mom, he has the mannerisms of one of our older half brothers—mannerisms he definitely could not have picked up the "nurture" way, since he was a six-month fetus when our father died.

As a result, when I went to select a sperm donor, I felt that I was not just ordering up a physical package—I felt that my child was quite likely to take after the donor and his family in much deeper ways. Like other women, I wanted the donor to be healthy and his family history not to include some of the health problems—like heart disease—my family has had. Like most, I chose donors who were racially similar to me—my choices ranged from a blue-eyed Anglo-Saxon like me to a brown-eyed, relatively light-skinned Hispanic donor—because I felt that looking like me and my family would be easier for my child. And I'll admit I was happy if the donor was described as handsome. But my biggest questions were "What is this guy *like*? Is he a nice guy? Would I get along with him?"

I wanted to know as much as possible about personality—the one thing there's the least data on, especially when you are looking for an open-identity donor. That's because, at least until recently, the only sperm banks that offered open-identity donors were the smaller, more progressive banks, which, perhaps because of their smaller staffs, offered fewer "products." Because I wanted to offer my child the option of contacting his or her biological father, I did not have long essays to read or the opportunity to listen to audio interviews with prospective donors. So I drove myself crazy trying to read personality in the tea leaves of the brief, handwritten donor questionnaires. Suddenly, whether the guy liked blue or red, pizza or sushi, dogs or cats took on great importance. On the form my sperm bank used, the closest thing to an essay was the donor's answer to "Why do you want to be a donor?" They had a whopping five lines in which to answer that question, instead of the half line to two lines the form made available for "favorite sport" or "How would you describe your personality?"

One donor, a musician and novelist (who I liked a lot but ended up not using) answered the donor question like this: "For two reasons: first, to get paid to do an act that I would otherwise be doing for no charge; second, I have been inspired by lesbian couples in my life trying to start families." He also wrote, under artistic ability, "I draw stick men." That was pretty much all I had to go on—two sentences—but in my mind, suddenly this guy became Mr. Personality Plus, sensitive and hilarious, a cross between Alan Alda and Robin Williams.

In fact, any casual comment about the donor by the sperm bank staff is often soaked up by the mom-to-be and can take on huge weight in the absence of more information. "They told me a story about my daughter's donor," recalls Suzie, who works for a big financial company in Nashville, Tennessee. "We always look forward to when he comes in, he's a good person, he makes us laugh, he's very outgoing." Those impressions meant a lot to Suzie, and are part of what she's able to share with her daughter. I had a similar experience when I was selecting the donor who turned out to be Scott's father. It was just before Valentine's Day and the client services coordinator mentioned that she had run into him in the coffee break room and they'd had a funny exchange about the holiday, the script of which I wish I had written down. In any case, he sounded charming and sweet, and she said she found him to be very handsome. Later on, when I was already pregnant, he had to leave the program due to an unexpected move out of state, and when she called to ask if I was interested in reserving more vials, she volunteered that everyone was going to really miss him. It sounded like he had charmed the heck out of the staff. Each little tidbit like that was a tremendous relief to me. If I couldn't really know him, or know if I'd like him, the fact that others did took on great significance.

For Anne, a single mom whose kids are half siblings, the personality part of the equation is highlighted for reasons similar to mine. One of her children has a dad and the other has an anonymous donor: "I have one kid who looks like her dad and acts like her dad." But Anne's other daughter's characteristics are more of a question mark: "I look at Lilly and I can't see what's me because I can't see what's him." She would like to have more information. "It's a little bit sad for me, but I don't think too much about it. Lilly's cute and she has a great personality, so it all worked out."

Lisa M. didn't really want to know much about her donor at the time she made the choice. "Back then, it was maybe a six-page donor list and there were no people of color. There was just one Latino, and he had really good health. That was the deciding factor for me," she says. Other than ethnicity and health, Lisa didn't think much about this man—he was just a piece of paper and the magic fluid that could get her pregnant. It would be Lisa's child alone, and she expected a "mini-me," she says, a child with her olive skin and the kinky hair she inherited from her Latino father. Toward the end of her pregnancy, however, she thought more about the donor—what if the child looked exactly like *him*? Neither happened, Lisa says—Mariah came out looking exactly like her Filipino grandmother. But the donor has made himself evident in other ways. Over the years, Lisa says, she's seen expressions or characteristics in Mariah, now age ten, that aren't from her or from anyone in her family. "I think, wow, someday I'm going to meet this man who's going to look like my daughter!" (Lisa's donor has agreed to release his identity to his offspring when they turn eighteen.)

For Jenny, as for many women, choosing a donor was an emotional, intuitive process, much like dating, and she chose a bank that was able to give her a lot of information to go on. "I wanted someone with a picture," she says. "As a visual person, I didn't even look at sperm donors that didn't have pictures." The bank was able to provide her with a childhood and an adult photo of her donor. "When I first saw his picture, I thought, Oh my God, I would totally have sex with that guy," Jenny says. "Then his profile made him even hotter—he was a firefighter and flew a plane and went to culinary school and quoted Einstein." She questioned her reaction—was this appropriate?—and decided that it probably made biological sense to choose someone she'd be attracted to.

What do the kids think? Danielle, a teenager who was conceived using donor insemination, was quoted in a 2005 article in the *New York Times*: " 'I hate when people that use D.I. say that biology doesn't matter (cough, my mom, cough),' Danielle wrote a friend in an e-mail message, using the shorthand for donor insemination. 'Because if it really didn't matter to them, then why would they use D.I. at all? They could just adopt or something and help out kids in need.' " (Danielle was one of the children of California Cryobank donor 150 who was happy to finally learn her father's identity—he was an anonymous-for-life donor—when he "came out" to his biological kids just before Valentine's Day 2007.)

Not everybody thinks more information is better, however. After her year spent poring over profiles, Liz decided she really didn't want to know too much about this stranger, after all—"I didn't order the audio interview or the picture; I don't want to look at my kid and see the donor."

"I'm glad I don't have a photo of the donor," Marcy says, "because I'm thrilled with my son, and what if I had seen the photo and not liked what I saw?"

## TOTALLY ANONYMOUS VS. OPEN-IDENTITY DONORS

Most sperm banks don't give you a choice—the donor you select is supposed to remain a mystery forever. But a growing number of banks offer the option of open-identity donors—donors who agree to have their identities released to any offspring who request it once they turn eighteen—and such transparency seems to be the way the industry is headed. Which to choose?

"That was an interesting decision," says Anne, who decided to become a single mom by choice after having one child within a relationship. "Coming off this nasty breakup with Roxanne's dad I just don't want the donor to be involved in any way," she adds. "Here's someone I loved so madly, and then he turned from Dr. Jekyll into Mr. Hyde." If that's the case with someone you know and love, how much more risky is it to make personal contact with a stranger? But then Anne realized she had to look at more than just her own gut reaction. "I already had a child who knew her bio-dad," Anne says. "So I felt it would be an issue, and I had to offer that option."

Jamie chose an open donor, and with her child's future interests in mind, she ordered all the information she possibly could, which included a childhood photo and an adult photo of the man. "I just hear so many stories about kids who are adopted and have a wonderful family, but still want to know about their biological parents," Jamie says. "I wanted that option for my child."

"It was very important for me not to use an anonymous-for-life donor," Shannon remembers. "My heritage and my ability to find out about my ancestry is very important to me," she says, and so she wanted that to be possible for her future child.

Likewise for Miriam: "It was extremely important for it to be an ID-release donor. I wanted to at least present my child with that option." She explains that a good friend of hers is adopted. "He's actually fine with it," she says, "but his sister has had resentment about not being able to know what her biological background is." Also, she says, her family history is obscured by war: "Past my grandparents' age, no one knows anything. They were all killed in Russia in the pogroms." Miriam wants to provide as much information as possible for her future child.

Kristen, a public-interest lawyer in Brooklyn who is trying to conceive has a unique perspective on this issue. She is the adopted daughter of a single mom by choice. Kristen, who identifies as African-American, was adopted at fifteen months in 1971 by her mom, a single white woman. Her mom later helped Kristen find her white birth mother, which was a bittersweet experience. The woman, a small-town schoolteacher, wrote her a note starting with the fact that she thought of her every birthday but ending with "please don't contact me again." Apparently, her having given birth to a mixed-race child out of wedlock at age twenty is something that would really disrupt her life if it were known. Still, Kristen was glad to have made contact with one of her biological parents and wants to reserve that possibility for her child. "When you're adopted you have this fantasy about who your parents are. I imagine it's the same for donor kids. My fantasy was that my mom was Jaclyn Smith, because she was the right age and hair color." In contacting your birth parent, "you get that debunked," which she says is a good thing. "You get confirmation that she's real." Kristen was also relieved, in a way, that her birth mother didn't want a relationship, because she had been nervous about how to manage that with her mom. It was a little sad to get the "don't contact me," Kristen says, but not really a big deal. "I had so many of my emotional needs met by my own mother, I wasn't looking to my birth mother to meet those needs," she explains.

Lisa M. grew up without her father, who left the family when she was very young, but it meant something to her to know who he was and have the opportunity to meet him, which she did at age twenty-one. So having a willing-to-be-known donor was very important to her. "Even though my daughter has a huge family on my side, I wanted for her to be able to find the donor, if she chose. I was always trying to be as respectful as I could be to her feelings."

Jenny chose an open-identity donor because of her years of work with kids from gay families, many of whom were the products of donor insemination. "The ones who were able to meet their donors were like, 'Yeah, I met him and it was fine,' " she reports. They weren't particularly focused on the donor, but were happy to have had the information and the opportunity for contact. But the kids she worked with who did not have that access were "mad or disappointed or felt like it was gnawing at them." Jenny did not want her kid to potentially suffer in that way.

Wendy Kramer is a single mom of a teenage son, Ryan, who was conceived by anonymous donor insemination, and she and Ryan cofounded the Donor Sibling Registry, a Web site where donor-conceived kids can locate their half siblings and, sometimes, the donor himself. Wendy urges single women considering motherhood through anonymous-donor insemination to think it through very carefully, and strongly recommends using an open-identity donor. "A lot of people going into it think it's just a donated cell, it's not a big deal," she says. But for the kids of donor insemination—and she talks to them every day; there are more than 7,600 members in her registry—it can be a very big deal. "To you it might be just a donated cell, but to the child it may be half of their genetic identity," Wendy asserts. "It might be easier for you to choose an anonymous donor, but it's not about you, it's about the child," she says. Parents, even single moms, can find the idea of this other biological parent out there very threatening. But the kids who want to find their donor are usually perfectly happy with their parent or parents and aren't looking for another one. "They're not looking for a dad to throw a football around with, they're not looking for college money, they just want to know where they came from," Wendy says. Before you choose a donor who will be anonymous for life, think about what your answer will be if your child challenges your choice, she says. Wendy has spoken to kids whose parents had the option to use an open-identity donor and did not, and some of those kids are angry. "If you had a choice, why didn't you pick a known donor?" they ask their parents. "Why wouldn't you leave me that choice?"

Wendy also notes that there are medical reasons to choose an open-identity donor and to try to get in touch with half siblings of your donor-conceived child. Sperm banks do not currently update the donor's medical records. "You get one snapshot of one day in your donor's medical history," she points out. "You don't know who got prostate cancer the next year or who had an early heart attack or any major medical issue. It could be significant genetic medical information. God forbid your child ever has a medical condition, at least you know the half siblings," she says. "I know of a few moms who have located the donor using information on his profile—just to locate him, not to contact him—in case their kid needs a bone marrow transplant someday."

Still, not everyone thinks having an open-identity donor is important. "Maybe my kids will hate me for this," Melissa says, "but I didn't particularly care whether it was an open donor or not. I didn't think it would matter so much to the kids." For Melissa, the bottom line was, "it wasn't going to be someone who left them." In her opinion, the kids would not have the kind of issues around lacking a father that come up in a traditional family if the father dies, divorces the mother, or abandons the children.

Some women are concerned that having the option to meet the donor someday is actually potentially harmful to the child, who may build up a daddy fantasy that then will be dashed by the reality of meeting a guy who just jacked off for beer money while he was in college. Liz specifically chose against having an open-identity donor, out of concern for her future kids: "In eighteen years, what if the guy's a total alcoholic or a psycho, and the kids are like, 'Hi, Daddy!' It's too random. I mean, it's not even like someone you met in a bar."

Kimberley agrees. "I felt there had to be boundaries," she says. She also chose an anonymous-for-life donor. "I don't know anything about this person," she explains. "I don't want my child to have a false sense of connection to this person." She doesn't worry too much about her kids' potential sense of loss at not being able to get any information about their father. "They can be sad," she says matter-of-factly, "and I'll never know what it's like for them—but everybody has something that they're sad about at some point."

Even for someone like me, who wanted an open-identity donor, the idea of that potential meeting is a little scary. First of all, it's hard to imagine how these poor guys will deal with meeting as many as thirty or forty kids who have such a strong genetic link to them and who may have spent eighteen years entertaining father fantasies about them. Maybe genetic offspring numbers one through five will fare well, but what will the donor's reaction be when a trembling number twenty-three places that fateful phone call? (Actually, Wendy says she knows donors who removed their contact info from her Web site after about five kids contacted them, because the idea of more was too overwhelming.) One of the things I looked for in a donor was someone who seemed like he'd be able to handle that kindly and gracefully, and someone who had enough cultural similarities with me that the chances of my kid finding a biological father who is painfully different from him would be minimized. I talked to several women who chose older donors because of similar concerns. In choosing a donor who was out of college, they hoped that meant that he was more mature and had spent more time thinking through his decision. "Something more than 'I gotta pay for my six-pack on Friday,' " as Laura puts it.

In any case, choosing an open-identity donor isn't certain to be any less anonymous than the other kind in the long run. If the donor dies before the child turns eighteen, the information the child is seeking may not be available. And eighteen years is a lot of time in which to change one's mind. "Just because he makes some sort of guarantee when he's eighteen and single doesn't mean he's gonna do that when he's forty and married and his wife doesn't know diddly-squat about what he did when he was in college," points out Robin, a senior-level computer programmer from Colorado Springs, who ended up with a known donor instead. Wendy Kramer confirms what Robin suspects: "It's no guarantee, and I do know of at least one case where the guy did change his mind."

There's one very small sperm bank, Rainbow Flag Health Services, that offers a third option, similar to open adoption. The donor is anonymous until three months after the baby's birth. Then the mother is provided with his name and contact info, and is required to contact him before the child turns one.

As you might suspect from the name, Rainbow Flag is a gay-owned sperm bank. Based in Alameda, California, it recruits gay donors (though it is equal opportunity both for donors and recipients, and in fact when I last looked, half the donors were straight). Rainbow Flag's donors often want to have some kind of relationship with the child. The bank limits the number of children to five or six per donor—extremely low compared to other banks. It's also unique in that recipients (i.e., women) are required to promise not to circumcise a boy child, a procedure that the bank considers to be genital mutilation and a form of child abuse.

Because of my extreme aversion to anonymity, I considered Rainbow Flag—for about five minutes. I quickly decided it was the worst of all possible worlds. Here's a guy you can't meet and you know very little about up front, but then once you have your baby he's in your life forever? He wouldn't have legal rights, but still—it could be a total nightmare, I thought. No way.

Rachel, a petite, pretty woman with short hair and a hip, artsy style, would beg to differ. She's the single lesbian mom of an adorable eight-year-old girl, who was conceived using a Rainbow Flag donor.

"It was quite a winding road," says Rachel, a university administrator in New Haven, Connecticut, that led her to the unusual sperm bank. Like me, she had wanted a known donor, and had unsuccessfully worked her way down a list of male friends, a process that took a year and a half. One potential donor took forever to reply, another waffled for a long time before saying no, and the last donor was enthusiastic but revealed he was HIV-positive. (There are now ways to virtually or completely eliminate the risk of passing along HIV from a positive male to a negative female by using expensive reproductive technology, but those options were not available when Rachel was trying to conceive. Even now, they are practiced mostly in Europe and frowned upon by the U.S. Centers for Disease Control.)

Rachel finally gave up on a known donor and went to a sperm bank that offered identity-release donors, but she had trouble getting the donors she wanted. Then some friends told her about Rainbow Flag. She liked the openness. She'd had many high school friends and, later, a girlfriend who were adopted and had longed to know their biological heritage, even though they were happy in their adoptive families. She wanted that option for her child, and as an only child herself, she really liked the idea of her child having half-siblings.

For Rachel, it's been a wonderful experience. Her donor turned out to be someone who had donated sperm as a social and political act, not necessarily because he wanted a relationship with the children. "He's not very involved at all," Rachel says. "He's super busy, he and his partner, and to get together you have to hassle him for months." Still, she feels it is helpful for her daughter to know who he is. They have photos of him around the house and see him from time to time. Is it difficult for her daughter that he doesn't want more contact? "No," Rachel says. "She knows that he's her biological father and that he's a donor. She probably thinks that's pretty normal." The result, according to Rachel, is that "she doesn't get wistful for a father." Meanwhile, having two biological half sisters has been a joy for Rachel's daughter.

Ironically, though Rachel has been completely happy with her decision, "If I had seen a picture of the donor or met him beforehand, I probably would not have picked him," she says. She would not have been drawn to his looks, and when she met him she found him to be a bit awkward and unable to relate well to young kids. But the daughter he helped her conceive is terrific. "How could you not feel grateful?" Rachel says. "It's just the most amazing gift." Her conclusion? "I tell people there's no such thing as a perfect donor, there's only the perfect child for you."

## WEIRD SCIENCE: CONCOCTING THE PERFECT KID

Shopping for sperm involves a bit of eugenics, which can get really uncomfortable—but is almost unavoidable. Sure, race and other physical characteristics are often a big part of the social selection process when people are looking for mates. But in the real world, personality looms large, and even what the person is wearing factors in. When you can't actually meet the guy, and all you know about him is his height, weight, hair color, and ethnicity—and his assigned number—it becomes uncomfortably clear the extent to which you are engaging in selective breeding. The echoes of Nazi Germany and its idea of racial purity reverberate eerily in both directions. "Since I'm Jewish," Melissa says, "I decided not to go with a German donor, because what if his grandparents had killed my grandparents?" Diana, who's also Jewish, asked the same question. "Do I want a Jewish donor? Do I feel, like Hitler, that Jewishness is in the blood?" Diana decided she didn't, and that the donor's ethnicity and religion were not so important.

But let's say you *are* looking for a specific ethnicity or physical type. Depending on what you want, your options can be limited. Minority donors are, well, in the minority. One of my exes is Filipina, and so we would have wanted to use a Filipino open-identity donor in order for the child that I bore to share her ethnicity, too. At the time I was looking, I noticed my sperm bank offered a grand total of one. Ellen, a straight single mom who's African-

American, wanted an African-American donor. "My [white] lesbian friends who were choosing donors were looking for things like music appreciation. They could choose between a blond who likes music versus a blond who did really well on the SATs. With an African-American donor, the pickings are so slim you don't get to engage in that kind of thing." Besides, she says, "I am sort of concerned that everybody who wants to have an African-American donor wants to use my donor."

Alice ran into the same issue. She (and her mom, who helped her pick) wanted someone tall—"I don't want to have short grandchildren," her mom said—and they wanted a donor with a baby picture. They also wanted someone African-American, like Alice, because they felt it would be "one less complication." But the choices of Black donors with baby pictures were slim. They ended up choosing a mixed-race donor with no African blood. "He's Guatemalan, he's Irish, he's all over the map," says Alice. But the obvious differences between her and her son's looks sometimes draw comment, probably more so, she says, than if he were the product of a racially mixed marriage, with the father there to provide the visual explanation. Alice tells of the time a Black acquaintance came to her door, looked at her son, and said, "He's mixed, isn't he?" Alice was offended and irritated, noting that the medium-brown skin of most Black Americans suggests they aren't pure African. "Who isn't mixed in America these days?" she asks.

Tauz, a massage therapist in New Mexico who was looking for a donor with her same racial mix, found one. "He's Native American, African-American, and French Canadian, and I'm Native American, African-American, and French Caribbean," she says. But in order to get the racial characteristics she was looking for, she had to sacrifice another thing she felt was important, which was to have an open-identity donor. "I would have liked that opportunity for my kid. But there aren't that many ethnic donors," she says, "so it was hard for me. It seemed like I had to make one choice or the other. Almost every ethnic donor was anonymous."

Kristen, who wanted a Black donor, also feels she's presented with a terrible choice. "Choosing a donor was hard for racial reasons," she says. "I chose not to have a white donor, because everyone would think I was the nanny and I think that would be an additional hardship for the child. But I felt like I had to choose between good health and 'willing to be known.'" Both are extremely important to her. "Because I'm adopted, it was important to me to have an identity-release donor," she says. She's still trying to conceive after two miscarriages, so perhaps there's still time to find a Black "yes" donor who has a clean family health history.

Carol, an African-American property manager from New Jersey, who was also looking for a Black donor, says she actually found Prince Charming. "He's the doctor I would have liked to have married," she reports. "He's stellar in the sciences, whereas I'm a more liberal arts person. We've got complete overlap of hobbies. He's tall and slim—with dimples! And even straight teeth without braces! He's a great addition to the family tree." Black sperm donors are so scarce, and finding such a perfect one is so unusual, that Carol actually came up with an imagined backstory for her guy's decision to donate. "When he was a resident," Carol is guessing, "he worked in fertility and heard people complaining about how there were no African-American donors, so he felt it was his duty to help."

Whether it's to match their own looks or to try to blend a donor-conceived child more seamlessly into an existing family, sometimes women do aim to do some biology-class selective breeding when they are choosing donors. Sometimes that works—other times, not so much.

Suzie already had one child with a known donor—a situation that went very badly (see Chapter 4). She decided a sperm-bank donor was the way to go with her second child, but she wanted her next child to be able to blend into her existing family as much as possible. "I have blond hair and blue eyes," she says, "and Christina's dad is Vietnamese, so she has brown hair and brown eyes. I wanted to select a donor who was somewhere in between." Suzie also wanted to select a donor with an easygoing personality and a sense of humor, hoping he'd pass those traits on to the child. She believes he did. "Eliza's got lighter brown hair and hazel eyes, and a skin color in between us," Suzie says. "She's laid-back and really funny. She turned out to be just what I hoped for."

For Ellen, a biracial African-American woman, genes didn't work out quite that way. She was careful to choose an African-American donor, even though her choice of donors was severely restricted as a result. "To me it would have been a rejection of the Black community and the Black part of me to choose a white donor," she says. But within that small pool of Black donors, Ellen found it hard to get an accurate read on the profile. Donor profiles are mostly filled in by the donor himself, but there's usually a brief physical description written by someone on the sperm bank staff. But such subjectivity is culturally based. "Is that a Black person saying that he's medium-skinned," Ellen wondered, "or is a white person saying that?" Finally, she just did the best she could, picking a guy she thought had "good genes."

The result: one of Ellen's daughters looks just like her, except that "she has the blondest hair and blue eyes, and she's really just white. She has my face, but I'm so thrown by her color. You'd think I had chosen a white donor." As a single mom by choice, that has plunged Ellen into an entirely new level of "What will people think?"

"What happened?" Ellen asks rhetorically, like the lawyer she is. "Genetics happened. I raised fruit flies in ninth grade, I know that. But personally, racially, it's just really something. I run into colleagues and feel like I should be saying 'Yep, I had a white girl,' because I don't want talk behind my back." These things happen all the time in the Black community, she says, but when a light-skinned child is born to a Black couple, everyone understands it's the luck of the genetic draw. It's different when everyone knows she had her choice of donors. Her fear? "It looks like I didn't choose a Black man because I didn't want Black kids."

Liz had a similar experience. "I wanted someone who was Jewish, and I wanted a donor who fell into my general looks category—I'm pretty dark, Sephardic-looking," she says. She ended up picking a donor with medium coloring, brown hair, and brown eyes. The results for her fraternal twin boys? "It's ironic. One of my kids looks like he's right out of Hitler Youth, with light hair and green eyes—though his features are just like my family—and the other is a redhead with very light skin!"

While obviously there's no guarantee what your child will end up looking like, Jenny, a single-mom-to-be, mentioned one practical reason to try to match your own looks—you'll get fewer questions about the donor, and your child may end up feeling less "other" as a result. That's what one mom once recommended to Jenny. This woman had used a donor whose looks were very different from her own, and so the father was front and center in everyone's minds. "People were constantly saying, 'The daddy must be this, the daddy must be that.' " Jenny took her advice to heart and used a donor whose coloring was similar to her own. However, there are some single-moms-by-choice who choose a donor to counterbalance any characteristics they don't like about themselves—tall if they're short, thin if their family tends to be fat, gregarious if they're shy—and some choose donors of another race to match the looks of a favorite old boyfriend, or simply because they think mixed-race people are beautiful.

## A FAMILY AFFAIR: DONOR SELECTION
## AS A GROUP ACTIVITY

Since online donor selection is such an alienating process, some women respond by getting their friends and families involved. "I know one girl who actually had a sperm donor party, and invited all of her friends over to help her choose," reports Kimberley. Though wild donor-selection parties may be the cutting edge, asking family to weigh in seems to be the norm, judging from the women I talked to. It's a way to try to humanize the process, making it a little less of a cold, anonymous transaction and a little more like, well, an arranged marriage dreamt up over the kitchen table, with Mom and Dad calling the shots. The newfangled technology seems to beg for an infusion of particularly old-fashioned social traditions.

"I really wanted a child who looked like part of my family," says Lisa S., the elementary school teacher from Milwaukee. But health was most important, and Lisa knew she was a carrier for a condition that occurs in the Jewish population—one that's rarely tested for. "In talking with the sperm bank and my brother-in-law, who's a rabbi, I decided not to use a Jewish donor." The final selection was a family affair. Lisa found herself drawn to one donor in particular, she says, and "I truly fell in love with the guy in his audio interview." Still, she shared her top candidates with her parents and three of her closest friends. "They all picked the exact same guy, for different reasons," she says. Besides, she ordered a baby picture, and while "he wasn't the cutest kid, by any means," she says, "he could be the brother of one of my closest friends' son." The choice was made.

"I read through the short profiles and then ran them by my parents and my best friend, and then got them down to two," Miriam says. "I was really torn," she says. "One of the donors is of regular intelligence but seems more social and personable," she says, while the other had high SATs and is a doctor. The same question came up that arises in the search for the ideal relationship: Do you look for someone just like you, or someone whose strengths counterbalance your weaknesses, and vice versa?

Miriam's family was divided. "I'm a bookworm," Miriam says, "and I don't have a creative bone in my body. So my aunt told me, 'Maybe it's better you go for the one who's social and outgoing and creative.' " Miriam's dad voted for him, too. "But my mom was going straight for the book smarts."

In the end, she left it up to chance, planning to order vials from both donors. "I mean, they liked them both," she says. Turns out, the choice was made for her—one donor was no longer available.

When Anne was looking for a donor to help her conceive her second child, she enlisted the help of her fairly conservative, Catholic parents, and it did start to seem like old-fashioned matchmaking—her parents really personalized the whole thing. "My mom read through the profile and said, 'This guy's too good to be true! We want you to be with this man—he seems like such a great guy.' " Anne laughs. "They knew it was irrational." Even her friend who worked at the sperm bank could not be totally removed about it. When Anne finally told her her donor choice, her friend responded with excitement normally reserved for a dating decision: "Oh, that's who I would have picked for you!" she said.

## DONOR PROBLEMS: ARE HIS GENES REALLY GOOD? CAN HIS SPERM REALLY SWIM?

Sperm banks test for a standard variety of diseases, and they generally guarantee the semen they sell has a certain sperm count and motility. But there are no total guarantees. Though rare, there can be serious problems, like donor-insemination kids who suffer from crippling genetic diseases the donor didn't know he was passing along. Or less serious but expensive and time-consuming issues, like the one I encountered.

My first donor was Mr. Popular All-American Guy. He was tall, dark, and handsome with blue eyes, and he was a well-rounded mix: on the ski team in college, plays the guitar, likes to dance and cook, has a degree in environmental studies, works as an energy consultant, and teaches middle school on the side. "He sounds dreamy!" my mom said when I handed her my top two donor picks. The other guy, who sounded artsier with a slightly warped sense of humor, was maybe more my type, but I decided it would be good luck to go with my mom's choice. (A few months later, I found out that two of my friends, a lesbian couple, had chosen Artsy Guy as their donor, which made me laugh—all the gay girls fighting over the same guy.)

Everyone else thought All-American Guy sounded dreamy, too, I guess—I had to wait four months before his semen was available because too many others were in line before me. Then I waited some more because I started a new job and had some weird midcycle bleeding. When I was finally ready for my first insemination, Dreamy's vials had been available for ten months. Dreamy was actually my first choice from my *second* round of donor selection. The first donor I'd picked had just hit his fifteen-family limit when I called to order vials, so I hadn't been able to use him. It had only taken that donor's sperm six months to cause fifteen viable pregnancies. So I called the sperm bank to find out how many pregnancies Dreamy had caused, fearful that he was close to his limit and I'd have to select an alternate donor again.

"One," the answer came back.

"Phew," I thought. Luck was with me. I had some time to get pregnant, and hopefully my kid would be one of the first from that donor, which would translate, eighteen years later, to being, say, number five to knock on the donor's door, instead of number twenty-five.

After three months' worth of failed tries, I called the bank again for the updated pregnancy stats.

"One."

"Why so few?" I asked, starting to wonder about Dreamy.

"Most of the women who are using him are close to forty," the client services coordinator offered. "It could be that; there's no way of knowing. And sometimes there's an incompatibility between a particular woman and one man's sperm."

Yeah, I'd read about that—you can literally have bad biological chemistry with a guy—but how could *all* of us be incompatible with him? I wondered. And all of us were having fertility issues?

After six or seven failed tries with Dreamy, I started to get really suspicious and called the sperm bank again to find out how many pregnancies he had caused in the year and a half his semen had been available. I'd recently chatted with my friends about Artsy Guy, who'd been an active donor for the same amount of time and who had not had a waiting list at all. He was at fourteen pregnancies, they said. And Dreamy?

"One," said the client services coordinator.

"Still just one?"

"Uh, yeah," she said.

"Isn't that pretty bad?"

"It's . . . unusual," she replied, choosing her words carefully. "You might want to consider choosing another donor."

I finally did choose another, a tall, green-eyed actor, again handsome, musical, athletic, and (as described by himself) "outgoing, courageous, compassionate, loving, loyal." Among the few things I know about him are that despite highly educated parents, he can't spell his way out of a paper bag (I hope my genes win there) and that his life goal is "to impact the world by artistic means," which I liked. Most of all, he seemed like a really nice guy, with a sense of humor and interests compatible with mine. For some reason, among the other identity-release donors available at the time, his personality stood out. I got pregnant on the second try, miscarried early, and then shortly after my miscarriage Green Eyes got me pregnant again with Scott.

What was wrong with Dreamy? I'll never know for sure. But, from what I have read, there's some semen, even if the sperm are plentiful (high sperm count) and plenty wiggly (good motility), that are wimpy, unable to hack their way into an egg. There's a test for that, but it's very expensive and, according to my doctor, unreliable, so the sperm banks don't do it. Dreamy passed all the standard tests that the sperm bank had promised they'd give him, so it wasn't the bank's fault and I had no grounds for seeking reimbursement for the hundreds of dollars I had spent on sperm and shipping, not to mention the thousands I had spent—not all of it covered by insurance—at the doctor's office. I had to just chalk it all up to bad luck.

Lisa S. had sperm trouble, too: "It turned out the donor I was using had some funny tag on the end of one of his chromosomes." She switched to a new donor, but then his supply ran out. Then her third donor turned out to have lower motility than her doctor recommended. "I tried with him but it wasn't recommended that I use him again, so I had to go back to the drawing board." If you're the sort of person (like me) who really gets their heart set on one particular donor, having to switch like that is excruciating.

## CRAZY MOMS: GETTING A LITTLE TOO CLOSE TO THE ANONYMOUS DONOR

Laura, who had twins by anonymous-donor insemination, didn't spend too much time thinking about the donor and didn't even order the baby picture of him that the sperm bank made available. That's because she'd read an article about single moms obsessing unhealthily on the donor, and she knew someone who she felt fit that semipsycho description—her cousin. Laura's cousin is the single mom of two kids by anonymous-donor insemination, and Laura felt her cousin focused way too much on the donor, creating a whole mythology about this stranger, based on the fact that he had Spanish blood. "Here's this Jewish girl in Brooklyn who has this son named Mateo," Laura says, "because of some man she's never met, who's probably no more Spanish than I am!"

"I think that's why I didn't ask for the photo," Laura says. "I think I was trying to avoid going crazy, because I think my cousin's crazy."

Ellen also feels like there are single moms who get too wrapped up in the donor's identity. "There are women who do kind of make the donor a real person in their lives and their kids' lives," she says. Ellen talked about women she'd read about—one who bakes a cake for the donor every Father's Day, another who has the baby photo of the donor displayed in her living room, another who went to visit the donor in California. "I feel like these women are kind of nutty."

Um, full disclosure: I may briefly have been one of those nut jobs. Now, I do see the donor as a donor, not a dad. I won't be baking cakes for him, or moving cross-country to live in his hometown with my kid, as another single mom did in an article I read. I found that pretty disturbing, actually. But the extreme lack of available details regarding the looks and personality of the guy who'd be the father of my future child made me completely insane. So in my desperation for more information, I engaged in a little sperm-donor cyberstalking.

It was at the very beginning of my anonymous-donor-insemination process. I had spent several agonized months studying donor profiles, and I had finally found one I liked best. He happened to be a performer who had a very unusual career and a distinctive physical description. And because of where the sperm bank was located, I knew where he lived. At one point I thought, wait a minute, I'm a journalist. This guy's a performer. There's probably pictures of him on the Web. How hard could it be to find this guy? I was unable to resist the temptation. And finding him turned out to be insanely easy. Within three clicks of the mouse I found his professional Web site, complete with details that made it one hundred percent certain that it was the same guy, links to articles about him and his family, the audio clip of a radio interview with him, and an entire gallery of pictures, many of them showing him smoking—which he'd assured the sperm bank he didn't do. White lies aside, I found the extra information incredibly reassuring. I did not plan to contact him or share the information with my child (though that last part might have gotten difficult over time), but I felt immense relief, having a more complete picture of who this person was before signing up to bear his biological child. Alas, fate prevented me from reaping the benefits of cheating: when I called the bank to order him up, he had hit his maximum of fifteen families and his semen was no longer available.

I'm not the only single-mom cyberstalker out there. Early in my pregnancy, I had coffee with another single mom, an apparently quite sane professional woman, who searched online for her donor for the same reasons I did, even tossing around the idea of hiring a private investigator when she was unsuccessful. (She eventually decided that was taking her curiosity way too far.) Like me, she didn't want to compromise the donor's anonymity in order to meet the guy or interact with him. She was respectful of his privacy and grateful for his help. Like me, and like many of the kids of donor insemination, she just wanted more information and a better sense of her child's biological other half.

It's hard to take the profound step of creating a life knowing less about the donor than you would typically know about a blind date. Getting that information by beating the system through Google (in my case) or through private investigation is not exactly honorable, and it's not fair to the donors who have only agreed to release a certain amount of information. "I think it's weird to hunt these guys down," Jessica commented, regarding a story she'd read about a mom who found and contacted her anonymous donor. "It's a real shame. This person basically did us a favor. The really unfortunate thing about women doing this is that it will scare away a lot of potential great donors." Indeed. In the end, I think it's just as well that I didn't get away with it, and that Scott's biological father did not have a unique enough description for me to even try to look for him. I suppose if I really wanted to, I could, but it wouldn't be easy and fortunately I've become more comfortable with the lack of info. In fact, once I was pregnant, I didn't think much more about the donor, and now I can't even remember some of the basic details from his questionnaire. It all really does seem much less important, or at least less scary, as time goes on. Still, I am glad to see that the trend in the semen-selling industry seems to be toward more information and more openness, at least for those customers who want it. And their future kids. According to

Mikki Morrissette, who just published her second book, *Voices of Donor Conception*, most children of anonymous-donor conception do want to know more. "It's not that they want that person to be their father, because they don't," she says. "They just want to know who they are, based on all of the things that have helped them to be." Mikki talked to many donor-conceived kids for her book and, she says, "I don't know many who are not curious about it."

## DONORS WHO DIDN'T INHALE: HOW DO YOU KNOW THE DONOR'S INFORMATION IS ACCURATE?

Sperm banks test donors for blood type and a smattering of diseases, but most of the genetic screening comes from the lengthy family health history that the banks solicit from the donors. Trouble is, there's no backup for any of that information. It's all basically hearsay. The donor, usually a college kid, may not know what his grandmother died of, or what genetic ailments his cousins have. And worse, the donor may want to conceal some of the sketchier details about himself or his family so that he can get that seventy-five to one hundred dollars per donation stipend, which at two to three donations a week for at least a year can really add up. Sperm banks say they are on the alert for such lies and, since the donors must visit often, they feel that inconsistencies and untruths tend to come out. But there's still no guarantee.

"I was really afraid of the lies," says Charlene, the mom of a four-year-old through donor insemination. "Every donor 'doesn't smoke' and 'doesn't drink.' " Yeah, right. Finally, she found a donor who sounded more honest. "This donor was like, I smoke a joint occasionally with my friends, and I drink when I hang out. I was like, OK, this is a real guy. Everything wasn't perfect, but I kind of felt his answers were more real."

Lying about smoking the occasional joint is one thing, but lying about family health history is quite another—and just as easy to do. Through my personal network, I know of one former donor who is now an alcoholic (Did he mention his family history of that disease in his form? Doubt it), and another who neglected to mention a lifelong struggle with a mild mental illness. And those are minor issues compared to other things a donor could "forget" to mention, like a family history of cancer or a hereditary blood disease. In the end, you have to hold your breath and put your trust in a total stranger. And remember the ancient rule of commerce: Buyer beware.

As frustrating as it is to have so little to go on, information isn't always all it's cracked up to be, either, and generalizing about someone based on a few snippets of information doesn't necessarily yield an accurate picture of the person. I had a couple of experiences where description did not match reality. At one Web site I listened to an audio interview of a guy who sounded perfect on paper, outgoing and witty, with rave reviews from the sperm bank staff—but in the recording he came across as totally personality-free. And when I looked at the adult pictures of some ostensibly "attractive" men at the only sperm bank that offered adult pictures at the time I was shopping, I wanted to cue the banjo music from the film Deliverance. OK, I am sure these guys were not mentally handicapped or inbred, just a little homely, but I found myself wondering what the real story was on the allegedly "handsome" or "pleasing-looking" men whose photos were unavailable. This is where my cyberstalking turned out to be reassuring. I'd been told the guy I stalked, let's call him Donor X, was handsome. Turns out he was, in an offbeat way. He actually looked a little like Johnny Depp. Seeing all the photos of him looking basically as described in the catalog made me trust the sperm bank's other assessments, though seeing him smoking made me wonder what other kinds of lies donors tell.

## FROM CLINICAL TO PERSONAL

One thing many women find is that their feelings about the donor-selection process change over time. You become desensitized to the weirdness, to be sure, but there are other changes that happen as well, and what seemed at first like such a clinical process often becomes a more emotional one. The most emotional part of it all, of course, comes when you hold the living, breathing results in your arms.

When Marcy began the process of choosing a donor, she felt fairly detached. "I didn't rack my brain too much about it," she says. "I'm not choosing this guy to fall in love with," she reasoned, "I'm choosing him for the physical characteristics." Marcy did not order his childhood photograph or his audio interview. "I didn't want to get too attached to him," she remembers.

But in the end, it seems, Marcy was not able to be entirely detached about the normally extremely intimate process of making a baby.

"The day I found out I was pregnant was the day I downloaded the audio interview," she says. She was nervous about it, having heard another single mom say about her donor: "I got the audio interview and he sounds like a real creep." But curiosity got the better of Marcy. "If he sounds like a weirdo, no one else needs to hear it," she figured.

Marcy was happily surprised to find a personal connection with someone who previously she had tried to just think of as the supplier of chromosomes.

"His favorite film was a French film called *Hate*," she recalls, "and I had just done a fifteen-page paper on that movie. He was really intelligent and had a lot of respect for his parents—he talked about his parents as if they were his heroes, personally and professionally. He just had a really friendly sound to his voice; it put me at ease."

Another woman who was very comfortable with the anonymity of the process found herself nevertheless very emotional while listening to an audio interview with a donor: "I remember tears coming down my face—just this connection with this person who could make my dreams come true."

My feelings changed over time as well. Like Min, the idea of getting pregnant and having a baby with the sperm of someone I'd never laid eyes on freaked me out completely at first. I hated the idea. It seemed cold and weird and unnatural—even threatening. A total stranger's sperm entering my body, and not only that, potentially creating a life. It just seemed wrong. I didn't like any part of it—not the anonymity, not the fact that my child would not know his father, not the medical nature of it, and part of me also recoiled from it viscerally. That's why I originally wanted the donor to be a friend—a man I love—and why it was so hard to give that idea up and choose a donor from a catalog, why I was tempted to cheat the system by finding out a donor's identity, and why it was so hard for me to switch donors when it was clear I needed to. I had spent a lot of emotional time "getting to know" my anonymous donor, getting used to the idea of him, trying to fall in love with him just a little bit, so that I'd feel comfortable welcoming his sperm and bearing his child. And still, I wondered, what would it be like looking at my baby and potentially seeing the face, the body, the personality traits of a total stranger? Would I be weirded out by that? Would it make me feel less close to my child somehow? I thought it would probably be OK, but I did wonder.

I should not have worried. I have a couple of childhood pictures of my donor, at age maybe seven or eight, and as it turns out, Scott looks just like him. But my reaction to that is very different from the one I feared. Now I see the pictures of this stranger I know only by a number, and he's not a stranger anymore. "I know you!" my heart says fondly when I see the photos. "You look like my baby!" My baby, whom I adore. So now I really do love the donor, at least in some small way, because he looks like Scott. And because he was kind enough to share such an important part of himself—his genes—in order to help me create the small miracle and the great joy that is my son.

# Trysts with the Turkey Baster

went out swing dancing one night when I was about to start trying to conceive, and there at the dance was a woman who was nine months pregnant. I told her she was my role model—that I was trying to get pregnant and hoped that I'd be dancing till the last minute, too. She immediately dispensed some well-meant advice: "Oh, don't worry about getting pregnant, it'll happen. Just go at it like a couple of irresponsible college kids, and have fun!" I smiled and just kept my mouth shut, thinking, I wish. It wasn't going to be anything like that for me. In fact, the day my baby was conceived, I lay flat on my back on crinkly paper, my feet in stirrups, while the doctor wrestled my recalcitrant cervix into view of the speculum and poked a thin plastic tube through, causing a small twinge of pain. "Have fun!" Yeah, right.

"It's kind of weird, doing it at the doctor's office," says Suzie, who inseminated at home with a known donor to conceive her first daughter, but went to a clinic for her second. The impersonal atmosphere seemed wrong for such a significant, intimate event. "You feel like you should have a candle lit."

Though conceiving a baby through artificial means may not be as much fun, it doesn't necessarily involve stirrups. True, some women hoping to become single moms end up using expensive and complex reproductive technology, like in vitro fertilization (IVF). That involves injecting lots of drugs to make your ovaries produce a bunch of eggs, then having minor surgery to harvest those eggs. The eggs and the sperm are thrown together in a petri dish. If that produces any embryos, a few of the best ones are put into your uterus in hopes that one or two will implant. Leftover embryos are generally frozen for later use. Cost? About fifteen thousand dollars a pop.

But that's the souped-up version of nonsexual conception. All artificial insemination really means is that the semen gets where it's supposed to go without the use of a penis. That can be as simple as having a friend ejaculate into a Dixie cup and then using another instrument—like a turkey baster or, for better results, a needle-less syringe—to place the semen in your vagina. Cost: less than one dollar per try.

Most single women without fertility problems do seek the help of a doctor, like I did, because shooting sperm directly into the uterus is statistically more effective (especially with frozen sperm, which, not surprisingly, is shorter-lived and less effective than fresh). Doctors can do a better job of timing the insemination by testing your blood hormone levels, by looking at the eggs developing in your ovary using ultrasound, and by having you give yourself a one-time shot of hCG, the pregnancy hormone, which serves to basically kick the ripe egg out of your ovary to make double sure the timing's right. Additionally, even if you don't have any apparent fertility problems, some doctors will want you to take drugs, like Clomid (a pill) or Follistim (a shot), to cause you to release a few more eggs than normal in order to up your chances of conception. (There's also a legal reason to use a doctor if you know your donor; see Chapter 4.)

Still, for the majority of single women who use fertility docs, the main process remains relatively simple. Sperm gets shot into you, same as always. It's just that instead of a penis, it's done with a syringe attached to a catheter—a thin length of hollow plastic. The type of catheter used to inseminate me had the rather sexy name "Tomcat," no relation to the celebrity pair. That procedure is called an intrauterine insemination, or IUI.

"People just assume you've done IVF," says Kimberley. "I tell them no, I just had sex with a tube."

Though Kimberley was joking—her tryst with the tube happened at the doctor's office—sex can be involved in artificial insemination, sort of. Some women—especially younger women or those who are not in a hurry—do opt for the closest thing to romance, and they inseminate with (thawed) frozen sperm at home with soft music and candlelight, making themselves come for good measure (some say orgasm helps conception). Or they do it at home more clinically as a way to save money, or because they are using fresh sperm from a known donor. The two over-forty women I know who got pregnant on the first try did so at home, using fresh sperm and a syringe. Candles or not, the basic procedure of introducing semen into your vagina is technically called an intracervical insemination, or ICI. These initials—ICI or IUI—are important to know if you're buying sperm from a sperm bank, because the prices and preparations are different. ICI samples come (no pun) complete with semen and cost less. IUI samples are "washed," which means the "dirty" seminal fluid has been removed and it's just the sperm, swimming in a preservative solution. (In regular down-and-dirty human sexual reproduction, the semen, which can irritate the uterus, is filtered out by the cervical mucus, so only sperm get in.) Knocking yourself up at home is cheaper and can help make the experience seem more human. But most older women who are using frozen, anonymous-donor sperm look at the statistics (it can take young, fertile couples a year of well-timed sex to get pregnant, and frozen sperm doesn't work as well as fresh) and decide to get medical assistance, as I did.

There are books that go into detail about the whole process of artificial, or to be more politically correct, *alternative* insemination. Unfortunately, most are aimed at heterosexual couples who are struggling with infertility. The books that are most relevant for straight women thinking about choosing single motherhood are the ones written primarily for lesbian couples, such as *The New Essential Guide to Lesbian Conception, Pregnancy & Birth* by Stephanie Brill, and *The Ultimate Guide to Pregnancy for Lesbians* by Rachel Pepper (who happens to be a single mom by choice herself and who did make her book inclusive of single moms, both straight and gay). The reason these "gay" books are the best bet for single moms in general is the fact that so many of the issues are the same—there's a donor but no father, and most of the women trying to get pregnant aren't infertile.

Your average woman, before she embarks on it, is not so familiar with the details of artificial insemination. Me, I had just a wee bit *too* much prior experience—and not just because of my years in the lesbian community during the "gayby boom."

Growing up, I spent most of the summer and many spring and fall weekends at my grandfather's dairy farm. My brother and sisters and I would help milk the cows, scrape out the milking parlor with this thing that looked liked a giant window squeegee, and ride down to the calf barn on the open gate of old Mr. Cowan's station wagon, our dangling sneakers making snake trails along the dirt road. We'd watch with fascination as he mixed up powdered milk in a huge bucket, stirring with his whole bare arm, his arm hairs suddenly becoming bright white. Then the best part: We got to bottle-feed the hungry calves.

In one room of the cement-block farm office that stood next to the dairy, the manager stored all the medical supplies. The broken-down cabinets were covered with flyspecks and brimming with dusty bottles of medicines and syringes and swabs. There was a small refrigerator for antibiotics, and, always, the big stainless steel liquid nitrogen tank in the corner. If you lifted up the lid and pulled up the handle, a cloud of freezing gas would start spilling out and you'd see the little glass vials of bull semen.

In the dairy industry, artificial insemination has been the norm for at least twenty-five years. Cows and bulls in this country almost never get to do it the old-fashioned way—farmers buy semen from the best bulls in the country, then often take it even further, flushing the ovaries of their best cows, doing in vitro fertilization and implanting sibling embryos into a bunch of unrelated surrogates.

When I was maybe fifteen, I got to help inseminate a Holstein. We herded her into a small V-shaped enclosure. Don, the cute young farm manager, pulled on a shoulder-length latex glove and threaded a long catheter into the cow as she struggled vainly to get away. I got to man the syringe and pull the trigger. Yep, knocked up a cow. Nice claim to fame for a city girl.

So, about twenty-five years later, there I was in the stirrups as the doctor pulled on latex gloves and started threading a long plastic tube into my uterus.

"I feel like a cow!" I whined to Dr. Kelly, and explained why. She laughed. "Actually, most of our technology does come from the dairy industry."

Tell me about it. Moo.

## YOU GOTTA LAUGH

Though I may have been the only single mom who picked up sperm on Studley Road and formally introduced her family to a plastic semen vial, I'm definitely not the only one who found something to snicker about.

"The first time, I tried to inseminate at home," says Kimberley. "My friend came over, and we were the Lucy and Ethel of trying to get pregnant." Kimberley asked her friend to assist: "You gotta help me!" but then said, "Don't *look* at me down there!"

"But I have to!" the friend said.

"Well, I'm not doing it, then."

"What does it matter, you're not gay," said the friend.

That did not make it more comfortable, and Kimberley broke down and did it herself. "I decided, this is ridiculous, I better do it at the doctor's next time."

It was crazy, anyhow. Her doctors were not set up to receive semen tanks, so she was having to ship them to her workplace. "People are so nosy, so I was having to come up with all these freaking lies: 'My friend is here for the summer and her son is on insulin.' " After she had her first child one of her coworkers put two and two together. "So, I carried your little guys over to you?" he asked.

The medical procedure tends to be a bit more controlled, but it has its wacky moments. Like administering the hCG shot—that's the hormone you inject yourself with to make the timing of ovulation more certain. You're given a small window of time in which to do it, based on when you're coming in for the insemination the next day. So suddenly you're the poster child for heroin chic. One time I was out with the woman I was dating and she and I had to duck into the handicapped stall at a Barnes & Noble so I could "shoot up." Fortunately, it's the closest I've ever been to being a junkie. Add fertility drugs, especially the ones for in vitro fertilization, and your home becomes a veritable drug den.

Barnes & Noble features in another woman's insemination story. Nina, who decided to use fresh semen from a good friend, says that for the eight months it took her to get pregnant, she and her friend would both drive to the parking lot of a Barnes & Noble located halfway between their homes and make the exchange, as if conducting a drug deal. He'd hand over a pre-filled baby-medicine dropper full of semen, neatly stored in a Ziploc bag with a paper napkin wrapped around it to help retain heat. (To work properly, sperm need either to be kept warm or professionally flash-frozen for later use.)

Catherine, a fashion designer who lives in New Jersey, is a straight woman who is trying to conceive as a coparenting arrangement with two close gay male friends. One Saturday night she found herself getting cozy with a syringe, a catheter, and a copy of *Getting to Know Your Cervix*.

OK, I know I don't have a date tonight, but this isn't exactly where I thought I'd be instead! she was thinking.

Catherine's first insemination was the strangest. "It's an odd thing when you're sitting there with a friend and you're not sexually involved with that person, but he has to hand you a cup of his semen. He felt very embarrassed as he handed it over, and said, 'I hope everything's OK.' " Catherine and her friends had ordered an insemination kit from the Internet, and Catherine had practiced using the syringe as instructed. There was one problem. "Water is not the same consistency as semen," she says. "I just could not get the semen into the syringe. I had to fight with it for the longest time. I called down to Joe, 'What do I do with your stuff? Your boys are not cooperating!' " They finally agreed that he would fill the syringes and she would take it from there. Still not so easy. The instructions for the kit, which included not only a syringe, but also a short catheter to get the semen closer to the cervix, had said not to press the plunger too quickly or the semen will bounce off your cervix and come right out. "And it does," according to Catherine. "I had to come downstairs and say, 'I think I've wasted your contribution.' "

After the first couple tries, though, the process became old hat. As he handed off the filled syringe, Joe said, "Call me when you're done. You want a pizza? I'll order."

Eva coped with the craziness by posting "The Adventures of Ava [her thinly disguised alter ego]" on the Single Mothers by Choice (SMC) Internet message boards. These short, tongue-in-cheek scripts for the film of her life include stage directions like "AVA (to herself—duh, she is an SMC)" and contain scenes of her grappling with the special fertility-drug syringe, shooting up on the sofa with only the television for company. "Ava plunges the syringe into her stomach. The show on TV in the background is now a rerun of *Dexter*, a serial killer who likes torturing his victims with syringes and other surgical devices, providing further encouragement and inspiration."

Min found it funny, too: "I was about to try an ICI and I was on the phone to the cryobank trying to understand how much sperm it was. My sister was with me, and she was asking, 'Is it like a shot glass? Is it like a thimble?' and we were laughing." (It's more like a child's thimble. The entire plastic vial, including cap, is the length and circumference of my pinkie finger, from the middle knuckle up.)

But Min's laughter didn't last long. She says she felt she had to try an insemination at home before she went to "this sterile doctor's office environment that I just couldn't wrap my head around." But she found the home insemination experience to be alienating, too. "Suddenly I had this huge tank that was going to be my baby's father. I cried a lot." While the semen vials are tiny, the stainless-steel tanks that hold enough liquid nitrogen to keep the semen properly frozen are about two feet high and look a little like unexploded bombs. There's nothing warm or fuzzy about them.

Julie, a government executive in New York City and a lesbian with a four-year-old son, had a good experience getting pregnant with semen from her known donor. She had just started seeing someone, and her new girlfriend helped with the first insemination. "It was romantic and fun," Julie remembers. "I thought it would only be a start. I inseminated twice, two days apart. One of the times Paul dropped off the sperm along with some flowers from his flower bed." The semen was in a recycled jar that had held minced garlic, covered with black electrical tape to keep the light out, Julie says. "He handed it to my girlfriend and me together and said, 'Have fun!' Another time it was a Saturday and we went out for lunch afterward and had champagne."

Liz reports: "My most classic moment was going to my doctor's downtown office to be examined, only to find out that I needed to go back to their East Sixty-third Street office for the actual IUI. This seemed fine until the secretary at the office reached out to hand me two tiny vials containing that mucus-y beige sperm, which needed to be transported to the uptown office. I asked for a manila envelope—given that I had spent thirty-seven years avoiding sperm it seemed an odd time to get up close and personal with it. She explained that not only did I need to carry it, but it had to be kept warm by being pressed against my skin—preferably in my bra. As I raced uptown on the rush-hour six o'clock train, praying no one would bump into me and crush the little vial, leaving me with my own personal Monica Lewinsky stain to explain away, I thought that this was *the* moment that captured the process of becoming a single lesbian mom for me."

Nicole doesn't mind the sterile doctor's office so much because, she says, "it's the place that could make all my dreams come true." However, she does try to make it a pleasant experience. "I love it when my inseminations are on a Saturday. I read the paper, and then go out for breakfast. Last time I scheduled a pedicure for afterward. Married couples have fun making a baby—why shouldn't I?"

## THE ARTIFICIAL INSEMINATION GRIND

My son, Scott, was the result of lucky try number fourteen. Eleven of those tries were at the doctor's office. Emotionally, the long path to pregnancy wasn't too bad for me. I had what I started to think of as fertility hubris—I never once doubted my ability to have a child. But I also had seen friends become emotional wrecks every month when they got their periods, and I vowed not to put myself through that. I kept focused on the fact that young heterosexual couples who are doing it like bunnies are not considered infertile until they've tried for a full year. Why would I worry about my fertility after just a few months of trying with frozen sperm, which is less effective than fresh? I reasoned. Still, I had fantasized that I would get pregnant on the first try, like a couple of my good friends had. After my third failed IUI (shortly after I was laid off from my job) I went to bed calm and stoic but woke up the next morning in tears. Also, as the months dragged on and on without getting pregnant, it became harder to keep doubts at bay. For me, deciding to become a single mom was like jumping off a cliff hoping the water below is soft and warm with no hidden rocks. So every month, I had to climb back up the hill and jump off the cliff again. It never got less scary. In fact, as time went on, it got more so. The doubts pushed their way to the surface. Am I doing the right thing? Am I cut out to be a mom? Is this a sign that I shouldn't do it? What if I have the kid and suddenly realize it was a big, big mistake?

On top of that, the process itself felt grueling. Each month, I would have to go in for one to three transvaginal sonograms (they put a condom on the probe—basically a long, narrow dildo—lube it up, stick it in, and poke around, looking at your ovaries). At the same time, blood would be drawn for my hormone-level tests—I had a small bruise on the inside of my left elbow for more than a year because of the continuous pricks. Then, every month, there were the two insemination appointments, sometimes involving a painful wrestling match between my cervix and the speculum, and one more appointment each month to talk it all over with the doctor. It was a total of five to six doctor's appointments per month, all of them early in the morning (nine o'clock at the latest)—a nightmare for me, a night owl who needs a lot of sleep. Weekend appointments were even earlier—I think I had one at six forty-five in the morning. I started to wonder whether the scheduling was some sort of hazing process to weed out anyone who wasn't really committed to motherhood. It became exhausting to the point where, when I had a brief, questionable-looking pregnancy that ended in miscarriage at about eight weeks, I was sad, to be sure, but my main emotion was relief. At least I was doing something different, and getting a break from the constant medical attention. Because of the pregnancy and miscarriage, there were almost three months in which I had very few doctor's appointments. Hooray!

There was a time, more than a year into the process, that one of the women who works at the front desk of my doctor's office made a slightly off-color joke. "Shhh!" said one of her colleagues, laughing. "Don't talk that way in front of the patients!"

The first woman looked my way. "Oh, it's just Louise," she said. "Louise is family."

I gave her a wan smile, feeling complimented but also horrified that I'd been there so damn many times that I was part of the furniture. As warm and fuzzy as it might be, does anyone really want to be considered "family" at her doctor's office?

I'm not the only one who had trouble with the insemination grind. "I am not a morning person," says Miriam, "so it's hard going every morning before work." Then there's what Miriam calls "the pincushion thing," because of the constant blood testing. "Which arm today?" she jokes. "When I had a scrapped cycle [due to not ovulating]," she recalls, in addition to the disappointment, there was relief. "Part of me thought, Thank God I don't have to go tomorrow morning. Before I started, I never imagined how exhausting this process would be."

Michele agrees: "Sometimes I think I need to hire a secretary to keep track of all my appointments. And I feel like I'm being siphoned for blood every other day. It's extremely hard. Sometimes I wish I had someone to go through this with."

Jessica dealt with the stress of it by hitting the gym, taking a lot of quiet time, and generally chilling out. "I decided I can't make myself nuts," she says. "Being nuts isn't going to get you pregnant."

Before she went to in vitro fertilization, Liz tried to get pregnant using IUI, getting pregnant once but suffering a miscarriage at about two months. "It was actually called something else because the fetus didn't come out completely, so I had to get a D and C," Liz says. "Can you imagine paying all that money to get pregnant and then having to have some form of abortion? It felt quite ironic."

Conception became almost like a job, Liz says. She just kept her nose down and kept moving forward, not really allowing herself to get emotional about the monthly disappointments, or even the miscarriage. For over a year, she says, "I didn't do anything but work, work out, and try to get pregnant."

The process puts a lot of stress on you personally, but it's also a challenge in the workplace—it can be weird and disruptive to be running off to doctor's appointments constantly. I got a taste of that, since I started the process while I was still working full-time in an office. It becomes harder and harder to explain absences. Nicole, who is still trying to get pregnant, says she started to feel guilty about that. "I've had so many doctor's appointments, my boss probably thinks I'm dying or something. The inseminations are at lunchtime, so theoretically I can sneak away, but inevitably some conference call is on that day and I have to be absent from it. I sent an e-mail to him saying, "Thanks for being so understanding," and he e-mailed back, "Hey, your health is our number one concern." Despite her guilt, she says, "I'm not going to lose sleep over it. My company has really been there for me, but it won't be there for me when I'm eighty in my rocking chair."

Too long a wait for a positive pregnancy test can drive women to increase their reliance on reproductive technology. After her miscarriage, Liz tried one more IUI and then switched to IVF, even though she didn't have any particular fertility issues. "I was feeling really impatient with the process and I realized that nothing about the process was normal anyway, so why not go all the way techno. That was a nightmare," she says in retrospect. The doctor asked, "How do you feel about twins?" Liz, exhausted from her year of trying to conceive, said, "Look, I don't care. I just cannot not be pregnant anymore." So they put in six embryos. "I go back and I'm pregnant with three." Liz decided to have a reduction, which is the term used for eliminating one or more fetuses in a multiple pregnancy so that the others can be delivered more safely. Right before the procedure she felt very sick and thought there might be another fetus. Indeed, she says, "one was a late splitter." She was pregnant with four, including one set of identical twins. If needing to have a D&C after the miscarriage was ironic, this situation with the multiple fetuses was in a whole other league. Since identical twins can have more problems gestating, Liz chose to eliminate those two. Was it a difficult decision? "I don't really even remember," she says—though since she described it as a nightmare, it must have been pretty tough to deal with at the time. "It became about the end game, not the miscarriage or the reduction or anything else. And I feel like the minute you have your kid [she has fraternal twin boys], the rest of it all completely fades."

Some women fantasize that the conception process is going to go quickly, and find themselves in it for a long haul. Robin found a counselor through RESOLVE (the National Infertility Association). The counselor happened to be a single mom who had gotten pregnant on her third unmedicated IUI at forty-four. "That's one reason I thought I could have a kid past forty," Robin says. "But it gave me a false sense of fertility." It actually took Robin ten tries to get pregnant, four medicated with Clomid, though conception happened during an unmedicated cycle with, it turned out, fresh sperm from her casual on-again, off-again boyfriend.

## THE WAITING GAME

Some women get lucky. With her first child, Diana only had two weeks to wait before she got her good news. She got pregnant on her first try, at age thirty-five. And with her second child, almost as quickly at age forty. But for most women, there are at least a few menstrual cycles of hope and excitement, then sadness when their period arrives on schedule.

I spoke to Nicole after she'd had four unsuccessful IUIs. Not being pregnant each month is "disappointing but not shattering," she says. She is concerned about what the long-term picture will be, however. "I read how women have been going at it for years," she says, "and that worries me. I know that financially I can only afford to do it for so long before I run out of money." It costs her twenty-five hundred dollars per cycle, out of pocket (insurance plans vary wildly as to what they will cover—best to check with your carrier, or even better, with your doctor, as he or she may have ways of getting you more complete insurance coverage).

"I think the fact that I hadn't told a lot of people made it a lot easier," Marcy says. "It was stressful," she explains—Marcy got pregnant from her fifth intrauterine insemination—but she feels it would have been so much more difficult if people had known. "It's hard enough to have your own constant internal monologue on the subject, wondering if every ache or pain is a sign of pregnancy or lack of pregnancy—add to that a bunch of people constantly asking you the same question and it can be enough to drive one batty," Marcy says. "Also, having people around who were oblivious to what I was doing helped stop me from focusing on something I had no control over anyway."

Eva feels the opposite way: "I think being secretive and keeping it very private is sometimes a necessity, but every person should have at least a few people to talk to. I had so many people whose shoulders I could cry on, and I have found that very helpful."

The waiting game has been very hard for Eva. Like most people, she started off hopeful, but after seven failed tries, she's feeling battered. "My first insemination was a special experience," she says. "Even after all the disappointments I still feel it. I felt pregnant, and I walked along the street feeling like, wow. I didn't touch coffee, didn't have any alcohol. I had such a feeling of gratitude that I even have the option, the freedom of choice, to inseminate myself. I felt empowered and it was exciting for me.

"The only thing was, it was difficult for me to do that over and over again. When you allow yourself to feel pregnant, what happens is that you almost feel like you had a miscarriage—when you obviously did not."

After a while, Eva changed tactics: She decided that she was not even going to allow herself to consider that she might be pregnant. After the insemination she drank coffee, even a little alcohol. "I tried different things in my mind, but in the end it's hard to really totally release the idea that you might be pregnant." So she still drove herself crazy during the two-week wait between insemination and the pregnancy test. "You're hypervigilant to every twinge in your body. 'Was that the embryo attaching?' 'My breasts—

they've never been this sore!' " Then the pregnancy test—or her period—would put an end to the fantasy.

"When I got my period, sometimes I would have to take off work for the day, and just walk around the reservoir," Eva says. "I always had some serious cries. I'd get filled up with this fear that I'm infertile, crying to friends on the phone, just devastated. And I'd go to the woe-is-me place: How come things are so difficult for me, here I am trying to be a single mom and that's hard enough on its own, and now I have this fertility problem, and if I had someone with me at least it would be easier." Eva laughs. "I felt that way even though I know through friends that infertility can be really hard on a relationship and can cause breakups."

Eva took solace in the Dixie Chicks' tune about infertility, with the refrain "It's so hard when it doesn't come easy." The song talks about a relationship that has devolved into constant fighting, about imagining the child being "a reflection of me and you," and includes the line, "I'd feel so guilty if this was a gift I couldn't give." As hard as it's been for her to go through it alone, Eva admits, "I felt relieved in a way that I didn't have to feel that I was letting someone else down." Still, she says, "The emotional roller coaster is hard. It takes so much out of you. One cycle I didn't try, and when I got my period I felt relief that it was just my period, and not a sign of the failure of my reproductive system. It's a hard thing when your body becomes your enemy and something natural like your period, you're dreading it."

In addition to fertility fears, Eva found, as I did, that the slow process teases out other fears. "I think any woman, whether she's single or not, has ambivalences about becoming a mother. And the longer you try, the more you have to confront your fears." Feeling momentarily defeated one day after half a year of trying, Eva posted an e-mail to the online support group: "Here I am thirty-four, after four IUIs, three thousand dollars in sperm costs later, some hundreds in co-pays, and all my hopes and dreams and disappointments, wondering how much strength it takes to carry on. I thought my age would be my ticket and now I just feel that it led me on."

After close to a year of trying, Eva is taking several months' break from insemination, to try to regain her emotional strength. But she feels like there's a silver lining to her bad luck. "I've learned so much about my body," she says, "and I've learned to let go of control. As much as I can create optimal conditions for conception, I can't control my body. It's going to do what it's going to do. Every month I've had to face that, and I think that's a good lesson when you're bringing a kid into your life, another human being who you can't fully control. You can create optimal conditions, but you could miscarry, you could have a kid who has problems."

Eva says she's also had to slowly accept the possibility that she won't be able to become a mother exactly the way she hoped. "Maybe I'll wait, maybe I'll have a partner who bears the child [Eva is a lesbian] and I won't have one biologically. Or maybe I'll sign up to be a foster parent, maybe I'll adopt." She feels like that's been another important thing to realize. She still hopes to have a biological child. But she knows that "if you want to become a mother, you can become a mother; just maybe not the way you wanted to."

## FERTILITY CHALLENGES

Many single women, especially the younger ones, have no trouble conceiving. Marcy was one of the lucky ones. She didn't even seek out a fertility specialist. "Because I was in my early thirties," says Marcy, "I just went to a standard ob-gyn and I paid one hundred dollars per insemination."

A lot of older women get pregnant easily, as well. Once I started using Green Eyes' good sperm, I got pregnant quickly, twice, at age forty-two. Anne had a good experience, too. "I'm a lucky person because my best friend worked at a sperm bank," she says, "so I knew a lot about how you did it. It was just a question of are you going to do it at home or at the clinic." When Anne went to the clinic, "they sat me down and showed the little chart about fertility and how it plummets in your thirties." Anne, who already had one child, wasn't too worried. "I figured, I got pregnant once," she says. Indeed, she got pregnant on her fourth unmedicated IUI cycle, age thirty-nine. Julie was almost thirty-nine when she did that first insemination at home. "I thought it would take me a year to get pregnant," she says. Two weeks after the insemination it was time to check the results. "It was midnight, and my girlfriend and I went to the drugstore together for a pregnancy test. It was positive. I didn't believe it. I got another test the next morning. It was an even brighter blue line. Then I went to the doctor for a blood test. Pregnant. I thought, Oh my God, I'm not ready!"

But single women, like any other woman, can face infertility, and that can be hard to weather alone.

Miriam started trying to conceive at age thirty-seven. When she was in her teens, she'd had an irregular menstrual cycle, but she'd been on the Pill since age eighteen and hadn't thought much about her cycle. She went off the Pill and was all set to do a couple of unmedicated IUIs to start with. But her doctor discovered she didn't ovulate, and there was a reason for that and for her earlier irregularity: She had polycystic ovary syndrome (PCOS), a common cause of infertility. The condition, which in retrospect Miriam realizes probably runs in her family, causes ovulation to happen seldom, if at all.

"I had prepared myself that the insemination wouldn't work," Miriam says of her first insemination attempt. "I hadn't prepared myself that I wouldn't be able to try [because there was no egg]." In a way, she says, she's lucky she was trying to get pregnant as a single woman through a fertility specialist, because she was alerted to the problem a lot sooner than she would have been otherwise. "I was so worried about my age, but this would've happened even if I'd tried in my twenties." When Miriam told her mom about the problem, they realized PCOS would explain the long gaps between children that were typical in her family. Miriam also turned to the Single Mothers by Choice online community and was reassured. "A lot of women who have the same thing I have do successfully have children," Miriam found out. She is now taking the fertility drug Clomid to improve her ovulation odds and two other medications to combat the PCOS. So far, she's had two inseminations and three scrapped cycles due to lack of ovulation or, in one case, a cyst that needed to be removed. "Thankfully, I have a friend who had been through fertility issues who has been great listening to me—she now has three beautiful children—as well as many other supportive family and friends," Miriam says, "so I keep trucking along."

Shannon also ended up uncovering a fertility issue she wouldn't have found so fast if she'd just been trying the old-fashioned way. When she started charting her menstrual cycle—recording the ups and downs of her early-morning body temperature, which shows when you ovulate—she discovered a problem, so her clinic had her use the fertility drug Clomid and progesterone cream, which can help some women sustain an early pregnancy. Luckily, she got pregnant on the second try.

Lisa M. was shocked to find that she was infertile at age twenty-six. After nine months of home insemination and five intrauterine inseminations at a nearby sperm bank, "I wasn't turning up pregnant," she said. The doctor at the sperm bank suggested she have a fertility workup to check out her hormone levels and the state of her reproductive organs. "No, everybody in my family's had babies," she replied. "It's not me." Lisa comes from a large Filipino family of "fertile Myrtles," she says, and she was certain she was one of them. As it turned out, however, it *was* her—for years she'd had a sexually transmitted disease that didn't present symptoms, but had been quietly destroying her fallopian tubes. She had a perfectly good uterus and nice young eggs, but neither eggs nor sperm could get where they needed to go. So she went to in vitro fertilization, and on her third try, at age twenty-nine, she was pregnant with her daughter Mariah, now ten.

Not all fertility specialists are good at their jobs—or the right match for you as a single-mom-to-be. Some doctors are opposed to single motherhood and some clinics are impersonal baby-making mills. After many tries at one large, impersonal clinic, Min got disgusted and switched to a private practice of woman doctors, even though the practice did not take any insurance. She discovered that she had uterine fibroids serious enough to impair her fertility. "The way the doctor put it was that I had a grapefruit, two lemons, and four golf balls," Min recalls. "In one month at that practice, I learned more than in a year at the clinic." But now she's paying everything out of pocket. "I took out a credit-card loan, and a relative of mine helped me out a bit, and I have a very small savings," she says. It's really difficult, financially, she says, but "I knew at hello that I was in the right hands." She had surgery to remove the fibroids, but was told that her uterus and tubes and ovaries are "picture perfect," so despite her age (forty-two) she plans to try more IUIs before getting more aggressive.

The process of trying to conceive is stressful enough as it is. When you add fertility treatments, the stress can skyrocket. Some women have very intense reactions to the hormones that are used to enhance fertility. Cheri used Clomid for her first cycle. "Man, that made me crazy," she says. "Hot flashes, jittery—it was a high. I was real chatty, dizzy. I was so sure it was going to work, and it didn't, and I was so devastated." Then for the second try, her doctor put her on a steroid (to treat her PCOS), and "that was really playing with my mind." Cheri had surgery after her second unsuccessful IUI, and then tried again, still on the steroid. "When I started my period after that third insemination, I lost it. I was on the floor of my family room, hysterically crying."

After that, she decided to take a break. "I ditched the steroid and did a lot of journaling, a lot of walking, and dated this really fun guy who made me laugh. When I went into that fourth insemination, I felt much more at peace." That cycle she used a different fertility medicine that didn't make her as crazy. And just before the insemination, she went alone to her church's candlelit Christmas Eve services for some quiet reflection. "I sat there and just cried. I had to come to terms with the fact that my timing and the universe's timing were not the same." Nine months later, the universe delivered her a healthy son.

Getting pregnant can also be rife with false starts, in the form of miscarriages or pregnancies where the fetus is chromosomally abnormal—both of which are more likely to happen the older you are. Debrah got pregnant on her first insemination at age thirty-eight, but then discovered the child had Down syndrome and decided to terminate. It wasn't a hard decision, she admits. "Before I even got pregnant, I knew what course I was going to take. My goal was to have a normal child and, however I got to that point, that's what I would do. I'm not strong enough, or the right person, to deal with a child with Down syndrome." After the termination she got pregnant again on the first try, and luckily has a healthy little boy.

For many women, however, terminating an intensely wanted pregnancy is an extremely difficult thing to do, no matter how compelling the reason for it. And it's all the more difficult for not having a partner to share it with. Same with miscarriage. I was lucky because my miscarriage was quite early and I had ample warning that the pregnancy was not going well. That helped make it a little easier on my emotions. But Nellie, an acquaintance of mine who is a single mother by choice, has had two miscarriages, both in the second trimester, just when most pregnant women think it's safe to assume everything's OK. Actually, the first time she had a miscarriage, the fetus came out when she was at a friend's house. Nellie was not comfortable sharing that experience with someone who was not an intimate partner, and she ended up washing clothes and cleaning up her friend's bathroom while still miscarrying because she was too embarrassed to leave the mess. The second time, she went happily to her obstetrical checkup and was told her baby's heart had stopped beating. To make matters worse, she then had to go—quite visibly pregnant—to an abortion clinic to have the dead fetus removed because, according to her obstetrician, that was the only place in New York City to find a doctor who was really experienced at performing the procedure.

"It's five A.M. and I was (finally) sleeping," Nellie wrote me in an e-mail shortly after she'd been told the second fetus had died inside her, "and then my brain decided it was time for me to remember what had happened, so now I'm awake. And guess what? I'm alone in my bed, with no one I can wake up so they'll comfort me, and no one else who's grieving right here with me (people offered, but it's not the same)."

As painful as infertility and other roadblocks to a healthy pregnancy can be, you just never know what's going to happen. Even if fertility signs look bad, the fact is that lightning does strike sometimes in a good way. At thirty-nine, Jocelyn was told her egg reserve was terrible, that she was going into menopause. She chose a friend of a friend as a known donor, only to discover that "his sperm motility was nearly zero," she says. "I looked at it under the microscope—there's a bunch of dead sperm and, like, three or four swimmers." Despite the fact that Jocelyn was on fertility drugs, "they said the chances of us making a baby were very slim." She inseminated with the dead sperm anyway, and found another donor that night, literally using a turkey baster to inseminate. ("Somebody asked me if it was sterile, and I said, 'At least as sterile as a penis.'" Jocelyn says. "He brought it over in a whiskey glass which I kept for years, and every time anyone drank out of the glass, I'd giggle.") Jocelyn felt guilty about having to replace the first donor, who was a really nice guy, but she didn't want to waste the opportunity. "Turns out I was pregnant with the 'dead' sperm," she says. "When I found out I was pregnant, I said, 'Are you *sure?*' They said yes. Then I called my doctor and he said, 'Are you *sure?*'" Jocelyn laughs. "It was really just kismet."

## USING A FERTILITY INDUSTRY NOT MADE FOR US

As a single woman without any fertility problems that I know of, I feel like a bit of a fraud in the waiting room, surrounded by all the couples who have been trying unsuccessfully for years," says Nicole.

Indeed, the thing about fertility doctors is that they are specialists in treating infertility. And they make more money, the more treatment they give. Meanwhile, most single women seeking fertility treatment aren't infertile. The medical definition of infertility is that you've tried to get pregnant through well-timed, unprotected sex for a full year with no conception. So, even if single women do turn out to have fertility problems later, most aren't technically infertile when they first walk through the doctor's door. Whether they're treated as if they are infertile anyway depends on their age and on the doctor.

Thankfully, my doctor did not automatically push me to do high-tech fertility treatments. Instead, she gathered information. She tested me for the hormone FSH, and my level came back very low, which indicated that I had a good reserve of eggs. So despite my advanced age (forty-one at the time I started) she did not suggest that I needed any bells and whistles to get pregnant, unless I was in a huge hurry and didn't mind risking the multiple births that can occur when you use fertility drugs. I wasn't in a panic, didn't want a litter, and couldn't handle the possibility of having to do a "selective reduction" (aborting one or more fetuses), so I went with unmedicated IUIs. Indeed, once I started using sperm that worked, I was able to get pregnant quickly without drugs.

Even though I was inseminating the relatively low-tech way, there were things I had to endure because I was seeing a fertility doctor that would not have been (and weren't) part of my home inseminations. Of course, it was ultimately up to me which procedures to agree to, but I decided to go with most of my doctor's recommendations. First, I had a hysterosalpingogram (HSG), where they shoot dye into your uterus and X-ray it to see if you have any blockages in your fallopian tubes. Most women don't have blocked tubes, but my doctor recommended the test because of the money involved in using store-bought sperm and medical assistance—best to know if there was a structural problem beforehand. Then there were the hated progesterone suppositories. My doctor preferred to see a higher level of blood progesterone than I had naturally, so she prescribed progesterone caplets to be inserted vaginally. It was like treating a yeast infection two weeks out of every month for a year—with waxy yellow goo. Fortunately, during the cycle I conceived Scott I had high progesterone naturally, so she didn't make me do it that time. But if my progesterone had been low, I would have had to continue the treatment for the entire first trimester to help ward off miscarriage. *Blech.* And of course there were those lovely human chorionic gonadotropin (hCG) trigger shots, where I had to pinch up a bunch of belly fat and stab myself in the stomach (though it really doesn't hurt) so the egg would exit my ovary on time.

Doctors are all different. Some are low-tech, don't use ultrasound or measure blood hormone levels, and will just have you pee on an ovulation test stick at home. My doc was in the middle, I'd say. More aggressive fertility docs will recommend the drug Clomid as a matter of course, even if the patient presents no hint of infertility. But there are risks involved with many of the interventions—while hCG is fairly harmless, Clomid is not. In addition to being associated with multiple births, it has been linked to cancer in several studies, so many doctors limit its use.

Some docs, like mine, evaluate patients based on their individual history and fertility profile. Meanwhile, other women I have spoken to have been told that if they're over forty, they must go straight to IVF, regardless of their individual fertility profile, and if they're in their midforties, they better use a donor egg, too (another five thousand to fifteen thousand dollars on top of the IVF charges). Is that really necessary? Maybe. Then again, maybe not. Statistics make over-forty fertility look grim, but women are not statistics. My two "fertile Myrtle" friends who got pregnant at home on the first try were both relative geezers—one was thirty-nine, the other forty. But when a 1986 study recently described as "classic" by the American Society for Reproductive Medicine looked at women who don't use birth control, and whether or not they have kids, it wasn't pretty. Of women who married at age twenty to twenty-four, only 9 percent remained childless. At age thirty to thirty-four, 15 percent did not have kids. At age thirty-five to thirty-nine, it jumped to 30 percent, and by forty to forty-four, 64 percent were childless. Of course, all studies have their flaws, but this one suggests that nearly one-third of women over thirty-five and nearly two-thirds of women over forty will have fertility problems or be unable to have a child. How that's interpreted in your individual case is up to you and your doctor.

"The doctors are kind of gloom and doom," says Kimberley, quoting the ones she saw: " 'You're thirty-eight, it could take you three years.' " In fact, Kimberley, who has a fourteen-month-old son and another baby on the way, got pregnant on the fourth IUI both times at ages thirty-seven and thirty-eight. Also, where she lives—Portland, Maine—"it's kind of hard to find someone who will work with you if you're single," she says.

Catherine's first fertility doctor informed her, "You are forty-two, and I'm not saying that you *can't* conceive. . . ." Catherine thought, Well, if you're not telling me I can't, that means I can! A friend of hers who had fertility issues said, "If you don't like what they're saying, go find somebody who's willing to work with you." That friend now has an adorable five-year-old. "I am so glad I didn't stick with the guy who made it sound like there are all these insurmountable problems," Catherine's friend says now. "It wasn't easy for her," according to Catherine. But it was possible. Through her friend, Catherine learned that you can't necessarily trust what the doctor says. "Some of the fertility clinics get a lot of funding based on their success rate, so they don't want to take on a bad risk."

I was quite struck by the experience of Nina, the thirty-five-year-old Baltimore woman who had to get pregnant because she was slated for a hysterectomy due to cancer concerns. She was using known-donor semen, and discussed with her doctor what the best insemination plan was for her. This doctor, a Johns Hopkins fertility specialist who stood to make hundreds if not thousands of dollars off her, depending on which procedure he recommended, told her that she could do it in his office, but that he thought she'd be more successful inseminating at home, where she could be relaxed. Based on what I've heard from other women, this guy was one in a million.

Some older single moms decide to get really aggressive because they're in a hurry, want to statistically optimize their chances, and don't mind the risks and hassle of medical intervention. That's perfectly valid as an informed choice, and one that many women I spoke to made.

Like Lisa S. She was thirty-eight when she started trying to conceive. She had six IUIs, then got pregnant. Her grandfather was dying, and she told him the news about her pregnancy. He died the next day. And then Lisa miscarried after eight weeks. She was devastated. She tried one more IUI, which failed. "I said, this isn't going fast enough." So, despite no real indication of infertility, she turned to IVF because the chances of success per cycle are much higher. She did not mind the risks: "I would have loved it if it had been twins," she says. The process yielded fifteen eggs, and nine became embryos. Lisa's doctor recommended that she only put two back in. "I am not a superstitious person," Lisa insists, but when she went home a plant in her kitchen that had never bloomed had three flowers on it. "Look," she told the doctor at their next appointment, "I'm thirty-nine years old; I want three put in." It did the trick, and she had a little boy nine months later.

Melissa ended up having twins by IVF almost by mistake. She was thirty-eight and had seen a TV report on freezing embryos. So she decided to have a "half-IVF," going through the process up to the point of creating the embryos. She'd then freeze them and keep them as Plan B, meanwhile still hoping that her new boyfriend was Mr. Right. She didn't tell her boyfriend what she was doing, and she asked a friend who was an obstetrician to give her the injections. Melissa's doctor friend happened to be a lesbian, and Melissa is straight. "All I could think was, Does she think I have a nice ass?" Melissa remembers, laughing.

According to the doctor, although ten of her thirteen eggs were successfully fertilized, the process yielded only three "good" embryos. If she were to implant them, the right day would be Mother's Day. That Sunday arrived and she was at her boyfriend's house. On a whim, she decided to implant the embryos instead of freezing them. "The choice was, a doctor's appointment at half past ten, or a ten-forty-five train to Long Island to celebrate Mother's Day. I called my mom and told her to meet me at the doctor's." Melissa had the embryos transferred to her uterus, and she and her mother went out to Mother's Day lunch afterward. "I was so sure it wasn't going to work," Melissa says. "I was sure it was gonna be like one of those dating schemes where you pay a zillion dollars and end up meeting no one." Turns out, two of those three embryos grew to become her twin boys.

As expensive as in vitro fertilization is, there are single women who actually pursue it not for fertility reasons but as a money-saving choice. Donor semen and shipping costs are so high that if IVF is covered by a woman's insurance, she may decide that the statistical chance at a quicker conception is worth the risks. But I suspect that other single moms may be railroaded, based simply on age, into invasive and expensive fertility treatments that they may not have actually needed.

That almost happened to Jessica. She was forty-five when she started trying to get pregnant. "The doctor told me I had a fifteen percent chance of getting pregnant, if that. He wanted me to go straight to IVF." But Jessica's hormone levels suggested that she was still perfectly fertile. "So I bypassed him," Jessica says. She decided to do unmedicated IUIs, while being treated with acupuncture. "The statistics for acupuncture for people who can't get pregnant for unknown reasons are the same as IVF," she says. "Why anybody would choose IVF first, I can't imagine, with all that pain and all the shots." She got pregnant on her fourth try, miscarried, and then had a successful pregnancy on the third try after that. At one point she went in for her insemination and was asked what day of the shots she was on. "I said I wasn't on the shots. They gave me a look like, you gotta be kidding me. The attitude was unbelievable." And the fertility doctor whose advice she had ignored? "He took credit for it when I got pregnant," Jessica says with a laugh.

Again, so much depends on your doctor and his or her philosophy, and what feels right to you. Carol had two kids already, and wanted to go for a third. "I come from a small family of two," she says, "and I always thought more would be so much fun." At age forty-three, she went to her gynecologist, who was also a friend, for a checkup. "He said, 'Look, I'm going to be honest with you, because I don't want you whining next year when you realize you don't have a shot left. It's now or never. At your age we're only talking about a ten percent chance.'" Carol chose to do IVF as a result of his advice, got pregnant the first try, but miscarried at seven weeks, and then had a successful pregnancy the next try—and she's completely happy about the way it all went.

Fertility doctors don't just have differing medical opinions; they've got differing social views as well. You may seek the help of a doctor who doesn't approve of your choosing single motherhood, and who may let you know it in subtle or not-so-subtle ways. Suzie, who lives in Nashville, Tennessee, ran into a number of doctors who simply refused to inseminate single women. Fortunately, she found one who would, and at thirty-six got pregnant on the first try, with no meds.

Prejudice against single women doesn't just happen in Tennessee. When Laura was forty-four—after two miscarriages from two different men who took off—she finally went to a fertility doctor in New York City to be inseminated with anonymous-donor sperm. "The doctor wasn't very good," she says—he was just using intracervical insemination (ICI), the same simple procedure she could have done at home. After her third unsuccessful try, Laura asked him if it wasn't time to go to the next level. "Well, you're single," the doctor replied, "so I wasn't going to suggest you use such aggressive methods." Laura was dumbfounded. In retrospect, she realized the man had wasted hundreds of dollars and months of her life (and her precious waning fertility). She switched to another fertility doctor, whose approach was totally opposite. He suggested, based on her age, that she go straight to IVF, using donor eggs as well as donor sperm. Her chances of getting pregnant with IVF using her own eggs were around 20 percent, he told her, whereas with donor eggs they'd be in the 70 percent range. "I was becoming desperate about my eggs," she says. "Every year is like falling over the precipice of a cliff as far as the viability of the eggs is concerned." In fact, when she was at the first "bad" doctor's office, someone said, "I hear Geena Davis had babies and she's forty-eight." According to Laura, the doctor and a nurse replied in unison, "Donor egg."

Their assumption spurred Laura's decision to go that route. "I decided I didn't want to risk it not happening, and I didn't want to spend eighteen thousand dollars on two more tries with my own eggs when I could spend that on donor eggs," she says. Was it a hard decision, giving up the biological connection to the child? "At that point it was just the next thing to do," Laura says. She did consider adoption. "I was horrified by what I found out, which is how prejudicial the system is against single people," she says. Many countries will not allow single women or older women to adopt infants, Laura says. She also had other concerns about adopting because of a relative who had adopted an infant who turned out to have developmental problems. Could it have been because of inadequate prenatal care? she wondered. Laura wanted to give her and her child the best shot at good health. "At the very least I can control the nine months of gestation," she figured. And she did not want to deal with the red tape of adoption. "Basically, my fear of lawyers is higher than my fear of doctors," she says.

For donor eggs, Laura simply went where her doctor sent her. That turned out to be a university fertility clinic, where, she says, "you really don't get to pick [the donor]—you have to wait six months and then they pick for you." There wasn't much in the way of description, either. "I feel a little disappointed that I don't get to know more about the donor. But I feel like I've done the best I can for [my kids], not subjecting them to my tired old eggs."

Laura's experience highlights the variability in the industry. Other tissue banks offer a relatively broad choice of egg donors. You can search an online database and find profiles, childhood photos, family health histories, audio clips, and essays for free. In fact, the amount of information you can potentially get about an egg donor eclipses what's available about sperm donors. There are banks that offer to provide a recent photo of the egg donor, arrange a phone conversation with her, or even (in some cases) set up a brief face-to-face meeting.

Laura's mother is an anthropologist who does not believe that you can predict things like abilities or personality based on genes, and she has been supportive of Laura's use of donor eggs. "She thinks the sooner you get that they're their own person, the better off you're all going to be," Laura reports. Still, she says, "I'm a little sad, not to have physical similarities. My boys are whiter than me, and I don't know what their abilities are going to be, though my mother says I wouldn't know that anyway. Either one of them is going to look like whatever they please, so who cares if they look like me. And oddly enough, they do have my grandmother's nose."

When Amanda, a New York City lawyer, first started the fertility process, she told the doctor she just wanted plain old artificial insemination. "I thought I'd get pregnant immediately," she remembers. She even waited a while to start, because she started seeing someone. But six months later, she was back at the reproductive endocrinologist's office. She went to the same New York City fertility clinic as Laura did, and was told the same thing: She'd better use donor eggs. "They sounded kind of like used-car salesmen," she says. "You have bad eggs, you need to get an egg donor. For a whopping twenty-five thousand dollars we'll give you eggs and just a few tidbits of information. We have a great donor for you, you have to decide tonight." She did not like the sales pitch or the pressure, and decided to switch to another fertility team. Turned out she had an odd-shaped uterus, which, in order to sustain a pregnancy, had to be reshaped using laparoscopic surgery. Not great news, but Amanda was so glad she'd switched doctors. "If I had spent the bajillion dollars for the egg donor I wouldn't have stayed pregnant." In fact, a year earlier she had miscarried twins from IVF—now she knew why she hadn't been able to carry them. Amanda had a bad FSH level (the indicator of ovarian reserve), but she nevertheless got pregnant, at age forty-four, with her own eggs on her second IVF attempt after the surgery. She's grateful that she did not allow herself to be discouraged by the first fertility clinic.

Jenny was thirty-six and did not have any fertility problems, but like many single moms by choice she went to a fertility clinic because she wanted to get the best bang from her frozen-sperm buck. She did not enjoy the experience. "It was such a factory," she says. "They didn't pay attention to the individual." Most significantly, they did not clue in to her single-mom status. "They kept saying, 'Is your partner coming with you? Is your husband coming with you?' After about five or six times, I was like, 'Could you read my chart?' "

Jenny's first insemination was a nightmare, she says. "I had heard from other women that IUIs didn't hurt, that you couldn't even feel them, so that's what I was expecting." (In fact, how much it hurts depends on your

sensitivity and on the doctor's skill.) She was also expecting that the procedure would be performed by the doctor she had chosen. "Instead, this guy
I'd never met, with no bedside manner, came in and was poking around in
my cervix for, like, ten minutes," Jenny says. "It was so painful." After the
painful and alienating procedure, Jenny burst into tears. Later, she asked a
staff member if her doctor was there. "Oh, yeah," she was told. "You could
have asked for him." Jenny asked to see him and then she let him have it.
"This is probably the biggest deal I've gone through in my life and you're
treating me like I'm coming in to have my teeth cleaned," she declared.
"You're disempowering me at just the time that I need to feel empowered."
Her experiences at the clinic were much better after that, and her friend who
was waiting for her in the lobby congratulated her for speaking up. "I bet a
lot of women go through what you went through but they don't say anything.
Good for you for kicking ass!"

## HOW LONG TO TRY

How long should you keep trying to conceive? Women have vastly different answers, depending on their philosophy, their stamina, and their
savings account. Some try for years, others try for a set period of time before
they consider adoption—or not having kids.

Miriam, for example, plans to try for three or four years, but only six
months out of any one year. "I'm an accountant," she explains, "I can't give
birth during tax season!" She plans to take her attempts "all the way to IVF"
if need be, but at this point wants to do what she can to avoid it. She plans
to go for at least twelve medicated cycles before moving to IVF. "You're not
even considered infertile until after twelve unsuccessful tries," she points out.

Liz tired of the process much more quickly. Toward the end of her year
of unsuccessful IUIs, she started the adoption process. "I began to ask myself, is this about my body having a baby or about me having a child?" she
recalls. "I decided it was about the child." Liz figured she'd follow both paths
and take whichever child came first. "I think that's why I got pregnant," she
says—"because I let go."

At thirty-six, Michele has been trying to conceive for fifteen months
with the aid of fertility drugs—"For me, having too many kids at once would
be better than no kids"— and has suffered three miscarriages. Now, finally,

her doctors are investigating the cause of her infertility. "I knew from the beginning that something was wrong, but they didn't take me seriously. So now I am relieved that at least I'm being taken seriously." She has started thinking about adoption, resisting it partly because of the expense. "If I have thrown everything I've got into getting a child, what's going to be left for raising it?" At the same time, she likes the idea of rescuing a child, and says, "To me, family is who you love, not necessarily who you are biologically related to." But now, the financial argument against adoption is becoming less convincing—Michele's attempts at biological parenthood are getting to be just as expensive: "My insurance coverage for this stuff ran out very quickly, which was a big shock. I've put about fifteen thousand dollars into this so far." She works at a small family-run company, which has been a mitigating factor in all this. "Working for my mom has been a real blessing," she admits. "If I have to go to the fertility clinic for blood work five days in a row and I'll be late to work, it's OK." Nevertheless, the process is taking a toll. "Financially I can't do this forever, and emotionally this is hell to go through with no end in sight," Michele says. "In several weeks, I start to have meetings about adoption, so at least if I'm told I can never have a biological child, I have this in the works."

# When You Know
# the Donor

As counterintuitive as it might sound, as a single mom by choice, it's risky to know your child's father. While you and your donor may not be a traditional couple, it's an intimate relationship, almost any way you slice it, and your emotions—and his emotions—can run as high as they might in any marriage or divorce. One divorced single mom I spoke to knew that instinctively. Lisa S. had a very good friend who she talked to on and off about being a donor for her second child (she already had a daughter from a previous marriage), but she ultimately decided against it. "I got very nervous about what would happen down the road. Being in a divorced relationship and knowing what custody battles and all the conflict can be like, I didn't want any part of that." In fact, under most circumstances a known donor isn't a "donor" in the eyes of the law—he's the father, with all the usual legal rights and responsibilities. He may be able to formally relinquish his parental rights, but that is only possible *after* the baby is born, and even if that's what he agreed to in advance of the birth, he has a right to change his mind.

Despite the risks, my first choice was to have a known donor. My baby's father would be a man I knew and loved, even if he wasn't my partner. He wouldn't have parental rights, but he'd be in the picture as an uncle figure.

Uncle Dad. He'd see the kids three times a week, or once a month, or once a year for a visit, with a few phone calls or cards in between—whatever version of "uncle" seemed to fit. My kids would be able to know their father, and vice versa—that was my bottom line, my priority.

I knew the risks better than most. Anyone with any sense in her head—like a lawyer, or a doctor—will tell you (and did tell me): Absolutely do not use a known donor. It isn't worth it. These sensible ones mutter darkly about the countless bloody legal and emotional train wrecks they've seen when known donor agreements go awry. Years of fighting, lost custody, pain, heartbreak. I knew all this, too, from my years in the lesbian community, where having a baby always means finding a donor. I was aware that legal agreements made before the child comes might as well be penned in invisible ink. They're almost worthless. If the guy changes his mind once the baby arrives, too bad for you. He's the father. The courts will grant him full parenthood, and possible custody, in the best interest of the child. That's a huge risk, and I wasn't willing to take it with just anyone. In fact, in thinking about a donor, my biggest question was: If the "uncle" agreement totally falls apart and I am faced with sharing custody and full parenthood with this guy, am I OK with that? I thought about it a lot, and there were two friends I could say yes to that with. I hoped it wouldn't come to that, but I felt the benefits of having a father far outweighed the risks. Plus, I knew three lesbian couples who had used friends as known donors, and so far their agreements were working out just fine. So, feeling romantic and hopeful, I popped the question.

First, I asked my gay ex-boyfriend, Xavier—we'd been a couple in college—and envisioned the tall, dark, handsome half-Latin children he'd give me. Xavier was a bit of an aesthete, a sensitive intellectual, the kind of guy who in college could be found pureeing squash for a soup or reading Rilke in the original German or scrubbing a speck of mildew off the shower curtain. In my fantasy, he'd take an interest in the kids once they were older, introducing them to the opera and discussing high art and literature, while I'd be the one rolling around with them on the floor, tossing them into the air, and showing them how to burp the alphabet.

Before asking him, I'd spent several months fretting over Xavier's suitability as a donor. Since I'd known him well for twenty years, I knew every last thing that was wrong with him. As with most of us, there was a lot. (I'd never have been accepted as an egg donor based on my dad's early death alone, never mind any flaws in my personality!) But on the plus side, Xavier was smart, sweet, good-looking, and, most important of all, I loved him. (I had this crazy idea about wanting to make a baby with someone I actually loved!) Besides, he lived in New York and was a slam dunk—he had been pursuing American citizenship for over a decade without luck, his work visa was about to run out, and he had asked me to marry him and (separately) had offered to be a sperm donor back when I was in a relationship. I'd said no then to the green-card marriage, since I had a partner, but now—sure I'd sham-marry him if he'd help me make a baby, though I didn't want him to do it just for that.

After my proposal, I sat back and waited nervously for his yes, falling more deeply in love with my fantasy children and imagining their trips to South America to visit their cousins. I'd have to learn Spanish, of course. Should I enroll in a course, or buy some tapes? Or maybe go to an intensive program somewhere? I'd ask my friend who had recently done that for more information about it. More importantly, who would we invite to the wedding? Did I have to wear white? Should I have my mom "give me away"? What would I tell the INS examiner about Xavier's toothbrushing habits? Would we have to get an apartment together?

After Xavier spent a couple of months thinking about it, I got my answer. No. He had a distant father, and he said he did not want to repeat that pattern. He'd actually had nightmares about it. He just couldn't do it. Besides, he wanted to get a green card on the up-and-up now, even if it meant he had to leave the country for a while. I was stunned; slammed. I had not even begun to see that Mack truck coming. Good-bye, tall, beautiful dark-haired babies.

After a month or so of licking my wounds, I picked myself up again and summoned up the nerve to ask my good friend Jim. My imagination geared up again as I pictured the medium-sized, cute, blond-haired, blue-eyed Irish brood that would result from mixing our genes. Jim lived all the way across the country, and since I'd known him more than ten years, I knew all the things that were wrong with him as well. But I loved him, too, and he was smart and creative and funny and musical and, best of all, Jim adored kids and kids loved him. I imagined my lucky blond children getting to visit him occasionally, laughing as he made up silly songs for them and taught them how to dance hip-hop and surf. This was good. This was maybe even better. These babies would be adorable and talented, full of personality. And since Jim's genes were even more recessive than mine, his kids would look a lot more like me than Xavier's kids would have. I had loved their dark hair and brown eyes, the look I'm generally most attracted to, but similarity was a nice thing, too—Jim's children would definitely have my blue eyes. I was psyched. I waited again for a couple of months, twitchy as a tuning fork, having no idea what he'd say. I occupied myself by going over the logistics. Jim would have to have his semen frozen and shipped to me, but first the sperm bank would give him an HIV test and then make us wait the standard six months while his samples were quarantined, to be released only when he once again tested negative for HIV. Not only would that cause significant delay, but frozen sperm weren't as effective as fresh. I'd better revise my plan. Maybe I could fly back and forth once a month? I scoured the Web for low fares and thought about the details. During my visits, would I stay with him or with my other friends in town? What would I tell my boss? Then I heard from Jim.

No again. Same "distant father" reason. Plus, he said, chivalrous straight guy that he is, he would feel responsible if I fell on hard times, and he did not want to take on that responsibility. I calmly thanked him, then I started sobbing the moment I got off the phone and could not stop for a day. I could not blame either of them for refusing. I would never agree to help create a child I would not then parent. Though to me, having grown up without a dad, a distant father sounded a heck of a lot better than none at all. But in the end, I knew I was asking them to do something I couldn't imagine doing myself. I also knew that this probably meant that I had to give up on the idea of giving my child a father, and that was most painful of all. I so badly wanted my child to have what I had not.

I wasn't in love with either of the men, at least not at the time that I asked them to be donors, but I was heartbroken nonetheless—and emotionally exhausted from gaining and then losing such a diverse group of imaginary kids. Then, shortly after I started looking into sperm banks, I freaked out at the lack of information and made a couple of other half-crazed attempts at a known donor, the wild grabs of a drowning woman. I considered a straight guy I'd had a one-night stand with—he had all the qualities I was looking for in these anonymous profiles, and I knew he was a decent guy because I knew him through friends who'd known him awhile. My intuition said he wouldn't sue for custody. Plus he had a ranch in Montana—maybe the kids could learn to ride. Why not him? Then I considered another gay guy, a friend of a friend, and was close to signing up for that—he seemed really sweet and had a lot of money that he'd be happy to contribute—but he kept talking about the child we'd be "raising together." Red flag. And I'd really just met him. Too risky.

Meanwhile, my mom, behind my back, asked a Republican golf buddy of hers if he'd consider being my donor. "I know three generations of his family," she explained. "And he's a really nice guy." Bob was enthusiastic about the idea, she said. I tried to imagine how my shy, conservative mom broached this topic with him and was equal parts touched and horrified. This is a woman who was scandalized when I took a college course on the psychology of human sexuality, because there were both male and female students taking the class—together!—and why would you want to know about all that . . . plumbing . . . anyhow? I talked to Bob—after my mom's conscription attempt, how could I not? We sat by the sea wall in Kennebunkport and threw big surf-polished stones into the cold, clear ocean water as we spoke. He had a great pitching arm, and he knew the name of the obscure sea bird that was wheeling about overhead. He was a nice guy, in fact—surprisingly sensitive. He was obviously trying to backpedal from a dinner-table incident several years earlier when, during a discussion of the Gennifer Flowers scandal, he'd dismissively mentioned "the dykes at NOW," not knowing I was a feminist and, more to the point, a lesbian. I really hadn't been in the mood for confrontation, but I'd never heard such language at my mother's house and I could not in good conscience let it go. My siblings had stopped chewing and were all staring at me, holding their breath. "Well," I began in my most cordial voice, gently setting down my lobster fork and turning to him, "I'm a dyke, and . . ." Bob's jaw dropped open, and my mom, who I was careful not to look at, was undoubtedly wondering if she could slide under the table and disappear. Despite all that, I did consider him carefully. I really, really, and I mean *really* wanted a known donor. But Bob really wanted children, he lived six hours away, and with the vast differences in our cultural and political outlooks it seemed like the potential for legal and emotional carnage was way too high. I thanked him very much, but said no. And with that, my known-donor dream was officially dead.

## DREAM DONOR

Unlike me, Jocelyn looked at sperm banks first—and that's what sent her searching for a known donor. For Jocelyn it was just too weird, deciding on a father for your child when about all you have to go on is hair color and eye color. But her search for a known donor had its challenges, too. "I had a lot of guy friends who thought I was an absolute lunatic," she says. But then she met "a friend of a friend's friend," and he was interested. "He was in his late fifties, was retiring, and had never had kids," Jocelyn remembers. "I think having a child was like his midlife-crisis Porsche." Jocelyn didn't know the guy and didn't have time to get to know him, she says, but "he was of a generation where I knew he wouldn't want custody." She decided to go for it.

"I was incredibly naïve and incredibly lucky, because, boy, have I seen some bad outcomes from known donors. Horrendous, nightmarish outcomes. But he was perfect," Jocelyn says. She traveled from Phoenix to Los Angeles, where he lived. "He was a charming and gregarious guy. We were going out to dinner and there was a huge line, and he started schmoozing the guy at the door, talking to him, and got us in," she recalls. When it was time to inseminate, the donor actually flew out to Phoenix from Los Angeles to hand-deliver the liquid nitrogen tank that held his frozen semen. "I think he wanted to be part of it; he was a very sweet guy." The night before the procedure, Jocelyn and the donor went out to dinner and talked about what their child might look like. "Oh, this poor child will have massive eyebrows and no lips," they told each other, laughing. Jocelyn inseminated one time with his semen, which the doctor had just told her was poor quality and would never work. She got pregnant on the first try. Jocelyn's brother, a lawyer, drew up a donor agreement. "If all known donors were like him, I would say everyone should have a known donor," Jocelyn says. "He would come every Mother's Day and act like it was a national holiday in my honor. He made friends wherever he went, and his daughter is a lot like him. I have to say I became very devoted to him." There was an occasional downside: "At times, I felt resentful and irritable because as an absentee father he was getting all the fun and didn't have to do anything," Jocelyn admits, but all in all it was a wonderful experience. It ended too soon, however. Jocelyn's donor died at age sixty-five, when their daughter was only four years old. "I wish my daughter remembered him more. And I get very sad that he didn't get to see who she became, because he would have been tickled."

Jocelyn got to know the donor's family at his funeral. They were a kind, conservative Jewish family. "He was the radical," she says. "His brothers thought he'd flipped, and they kept trying to get him to make an honest woman out of me." While the donor's family didn't understand the agreement, they were warm and hospitable. "As somebody said to me, they're a 'do the right thing' family." But the differences in culture, in addition to the differences in age—Jocelyn's daughter was in a generation by herself—have made it so Jocelyn and her daughter have not kept in close touch with the donor's family. Jocelyn and her daughter stayed with his relatives for the funeral, in a home where they kept kosher. "I was trying really hard to follow all the rules, but I don't know all the rules. At one point I put a sweet potato in a pan and it was the wrong pan [she thinks she may have been cooking it with butter in a pan meant only for meat], and they spent the next hour trying to decide whether they needed to throw away the pan. I felt like I blundered my way through everything."

Jocelyn admits she got "extraordinarily lucky" with her known donor. "Today, with as little information as I had about her father, I probably would go with ID-release," she says—in other words, she'd select an anonymous donor from a sperm bank.

## DIFFERENT WAYS OF FINDING KNOWN DONORS

Many women end up asking old boyfriends to be their donors, as I did. Others ask close friends, or find a friend of a friend. And, at least in the gay community, some actually find a known donor through a support group—usually gay men and lesbians looking to coparent. Some straight women in casual relationships end up asking their current boyfriend to be the donor, though that creates a situation ripe for misunderstanding and conflict if both parties are not being completely honest—with themselves and with each other—about their expectations and intentions. None of the women who I talked to who went with known donors used a doctor for the insemination. Unless there's a geographical issue or a fertility problem, it's not necessary from a reproductive point of view. But it may be an extremely important legal consideration, depending on what your agreement with the donor is and what state you live in. In some states, using a doctor as an intermediary will help prove that the donor is just a donor, not a dad, while if you don't use a doctor, the donor is legally a full parent with all the usual rights and responsibilities. The problem with using a doctor, though, is that if the donor is not your husband or partner, the doctor will not want to inseminate you with fresh semen for fear of being held liable if you contract HIV or some other sexually transmitted disease. The doctor will want to freeze the semen, wait six months, and then retest your donor for HIV. Problem with that is, you lose six months and you end up using frozen semen, which is less effective than fresh.

Nina asked a close gay friend to be her donor. "Basically, this was the cheapest way," she admits. "I sent him an e-mail and he called me right away. He was thrilled, because he's gay and he knows he won't have kids of his own—not necessarily because he's gay but because he's an actor and doesn't make a lot of money or have a consistent schedule." They agreed that he would not be a parent, but that he'd spend time with the baby one weekend a month. "For him, he feels like he gets to have the best of both worlds," says Nina. "He gets to see the child without being responsible financially." Nina feels like she's getting a good deal, too: "Of all the guys I'd dated or was friends with, he had the gentlest spirit. He was creative and smart."

Robin, meanwhile, asked the guy who she was casually dating to be her known donor. "He was sort of iffy about the idea," she says. "He was bemoaning his genetics, and when it came to the time of the month that mattered, he was playing games [like pulling his penis out before ejaculating]." Robin's boyfriend came to a couple of her fertility counseling sessions, but didn't want to codify anything. *"Que será, será,"* he'd say, and he refused to put any agreement down on paper. Robin says her logical side told her to go with an anonymous donor, "like all the other logical ladies. But my heart said, I want a known donor." So Robin decided to play it both ways. She picked a sperm donor, going for someone totally different from herself. "I'm a computer person, very logical," she says, "so I went creative—animation people, people who can draw." She went to a fertility doctor for inseminations with the anonymous donor sperm. Meanwhile, she still saw her computer-geek boyfriend from time to time. "I had him around monthly if he was feeling up to it. Sometimes he did, sometimes he didn't."

It took Robin ten tries to get pregnant, and four of the tries were medicated with Clomid to make her produce more eggs. But her last try was just a natural, unmedicated cycle. "I was supposed to have a rest cycle and they were looking at me for IVF, but I had a huge old luscious follicle and so the nurse and I decided I should take advantage of it." They gave Robin an hCG shot to trigger ovulation, and she had sex with her boyfriend right after. Then she had an intrauterine insemination two days later, when ovulation was scheduled to occur. She got pregnant. But who was the father? Robin had no idea. "I didn't find out until we checked the blood type when the kid was born." Robin and her boyfriend did put together a donor agreement after the fact. "It basically says that I won't ask for money and he won't sue for custody. But known-donor agreements are sort of bogus anyway," says Robin. She knows they can be disregarded in court. "Either my heart or my logic was gonna win." And Robin went with her heart. "You kind of want a father, in some sense. My kid knows he has a father, and I can look at my kid's toes and say, 'Those are his father's toes.' It's kind of neat. It's that sense of belonging and that he has two sides to his family."

It isn't all cute toes. There are significant legal ramifications to being a single mom with a known donor. "There's a lot of trickiness with a known donor, because he could sue for custody," Robin admits. "But if you can communicate with the guy, I don't know that you'll have problems. If you keep the lines of communication open, you can tell when things are going sour." And you can work to squelch a battle before it becomes a war. She feels like choosing a known donor gets an undeservedly bad rap. "I only know of one woman who had to go through being sued for visitation," says Robin, who is active in the national online community of Single Mothers by Choice and so is in communication with hundreds of single moms. "I tend to think that folks who did anonymous donor insemination think having a known donor is a lot scarier than it really is."

In fact, Robin takes a very pro-known-donor stance. While she recognizes that there are some valid reasons to choose an anonymous donor, she gets impatient when she hears women list the risks of a known donor. You're just a bunch of control freaks, she thinks. She wonders if women who choose anonymous donor sperm are trying to control their parenting experience at the expense of their children. "Those of us who choose to be single moms are usually at the pinnacle of success, and we did that by orchestrating our rise—and that's great," Robin points out. "But you got to let up on that and let someone else into your life, because the kid should know his father." She feels that women who choose known donors are taking a risk in order that their children may benefit. "We see that the kid knowing his father is worth the torment of thinking you might get pulled into court."

## WHY SOME WOMEN DECIDE AGAINST KNOWING THEIR CHILD'S FATHER

While Robin strongly supports using known donors and others, like Mikki Morrissette, also favor it, there are many single moms who feel the risks just aren't worth it. "Once you have human beings, personal feelings come into play," says Marcy. "My parents divorced when I was thirteen. I have so many memories of them fighting." She did not want to do that to her child, and having a baby with a known donor seemed like it was risking that as a possibility. A donor may agree to one thing before the fact, but change his mind later. "Who knows how he's going to feel when the baby is born?" Marcy asks. And who knows how she will feel? "What if I'm up all night with this crying baby, and I know the donor. Will I feel like he should be there to help?"

Kimberley believes a known donor would be too much of a mixed message for the child. When Kimberley let people know she was pregnant, "everyone wanted in on helping. Men came out of the woodwork." But she didn't feel that was right. "I never wanted to look at a child that I love and say, 'I didn't think he'd be OK for a husband for me, but for your father for the rest of your life I thought he was fine.' "

Jenny, who is nineteen weeks pregnant, thought about finding a known donor "for about five minutes," she remembers. Her parents divorced when she was a teenager and there was a protracted legal battle around custody and other issues regarding her and her siblings. That was hard on her, and it's something she wants to protect her future child from. "I don't want there to be a risk of putting my child through any kind of battle," she declares. Choosing an anonymous donor felt safer, both emotionally and legally. Additionally, Jenny still hopes to find a husband and a father for her kid. Guys don't like it when there's another guy around, a friend of hers pointed out to her. "I want there to be space in my life for the man to come into," says Jenny.

Other single moms I spoke to would have liked to have used a known

donor, but, as for me, it wasn't destined to happen that way. Jessica had originally wanted to use a known donor, "a gay friend of many years," but it didn't
work out. She liked the idea of a known donor because it would give her
child "the most resources possible." She felt the donor could be as involved
or uninvolved as he wanted. "It would make my life more complicated, and
I knew that, but it would give my child much more to draw from," Jessica
felt. Unfortunately, the donor decided it was too much for him to consider,
and Jessica ended up using an anonymous sperm-bank donor.

## KNOWN DONOR FROM HELL

Suzie might have agreed with Robin that taking the risk of being sued for
custody was worth it so her child could have a dad—until she lost that
particular game of chance. She chose a known donor, got pulled into court,
he was awarded partial custody, and now it's not only her but also her daughter who suffers the torment. Another single mother I talked to said she rejected the idea of using a known donor because, given the risks involved, she
felt it would be "a Lifetime movie in the making." Unfortunately, Suzie's life
is that made-for-TV movie.

Suzie chose a known donor for all the right reasons. It was supposed to
be a positive thing for her kid. "Even if I wasn't married, I thought it would
be better to have a father figure, at least," Suzie says. So she asked a guy she'd
been dating on and off to be a donor. It was at a point they'd decided to be
just friends. "I thought he seemed like a nice person and we'd been friends
for a while," Suzie recalls. The guy agreed, and they informally wrote down
all the specifics. "No legal custody, no child support," Suzie said they agreed
regarding his role. "He'd be kind of the father figure, kind of like if he were
my brother, so the child, especially if it turned out to be a boy, would have
a male role model."

It all looked good—until Suzie got pregnant. "Suddenly he wanted more,
he wanted to date, he wanted to get married," Suzie remembers. Suzie didn't.
When she gave birth, Suzie says, "I ended up having to be at the hospital
under an assumed name because of his threats." The situation escalated once
their baby girl was born. "He threatened to kidnap her. 'I'm going to take her
away from you unless you marry me,' he said." Suzie didn't marry him, so the
ex-boyfriend-donor made good on his threat and took his daughter—the

legal way. They now have joint custody. The donor has their daughter on first, third, and fifth weekends, and summers. And his threatening behavior now is directed toward the little girl. "He's a very angry man about the fact that I didn't want to pursue things," says Suzie. "He's been told to go to counseling and stuff," she adds, but the anger continues. "I think you see the signs afterward," she says. "For example, a dry cleaner lost his shirt. They paid him for the loss, but he still kept on going back for years afterward, harassing them to find the shirt: 'I know you paid me, but I still want my shirt.' The dry cleaner finally called the police, but he still kept going back. I was disturbed by that, and told him I was concerned he'd do something like that with me. And he said, 'No, I would never do anything like that to you.' " Suzie wishes she had paid more attention to such red flags.

The girl, Christina, is now ten years old. "Christina cries before she goes," Suzie says. "She cries, she shakes, she just doesn't know what he's going to do." The supposed reasons for his anger are so absurd as to almost be funny. Recently, it's earrings. "I got her ears pierced," Suzie explains. "We had a legal agreement that she could have her ears pierced at age ten. So she got her ears pierced." According to the health-care provider's guidelines, she was supposed to keep the initial gold posts in for four to six weeks. But the donor, her father, wanted them to stay in for a year. The judge said that she could follow the health-care guidelines. But that didn't change her father's mind. "So every time she changes her earrings out at his house, he punishes her, withholds food, screams and yells, puts her in the closet." Every night before Christina goes to sleep, she cries. "She's afraid if she changes her earrings, what he might do to her animals over there. We talk about what to do, who to call if he were ever to hit her. This is the kind of stuff we have to practice because she's so afraid of him." Suzie has reported these things to the family court, to no avail. "They don't recognize emotional abuse as much as physical abuse," Suzie says. "He is so bad, she is starting to have a bad view of men. I've had to start saying, no, this kind of thing is very rare, men can be very nice."

There isn't much Suzie can do besides attempt to help keep Christina's spirits up. "I try to do little things, write little notes to get her through this. I gave her the footprints in the sand poem [in which a man who thought he'd been abandoned by God in his darkest hour realizes that God was actually carrying him], to try to give her a more spiritual perspective. I tell her she'll have more sympathy for others when she grows up, and that she'll be a stronger person for it." Suzie originally chose a known donor so that her daughter could have a relationship with her father. But what does Suzie think will happen when Christina turns eighteen, or if the judge changes the custody agreement? "I don't think she'll have anything to do with him."

"I made a huge mistake," Suzie says. "Based on what I've learned, I think using an anonymous donor and then finding a friend who's a father figure is a better bet for everyone." That's what Suzie did to have her younger daughter, Eliza, who's now eight. "Christina says, 'Eliza has the perfect life because she doesn't have to go,'" Suzie reports.

Known-donor issues don't always hit that level of insanity, but using a past or present sex partner as a donor can be a bad choice—there can be too many muddled emotions involved, never mind that he's legally the parent. When Amy was thirty-seven, and feeling like she'd never find someone to raise a child with, she hooked up with an old boyfriend. "I told him we need to take precautions, and he said, 'We do?'" So they didn't. "In my head I wanted a baby, but didn't need someone to raise a baby with," says Amy. In any case, this guy was not husband material to her mind. Meanwhile, Amy says, "He was thinking, if I get her pregnant she'll marry me."

She got pregnant—but she didn't want to marry him. "I want you to be in his life," she says she told him, "but I don't see getting married just because of the baby; we're too unstable." Having a child with this man was a disaster from the beginning, Amy recalls. "He wanted to be a dad more than anything, he wanted to be a part of the pregnancy, he wanted to see me growing, he just wanted me," Amy says. "And I just kept pushing him away. He was very angry. It was unpleasant the entire time I was pregnant." The conflict continued through their son's birth and short life, and after his death from SIDS, his two parents were left alone in their grief, with so many hard feelings between then that they were unable to comfort each other and help each other cope.

## THE DONOR AS COPARENT

Julie had a son with a lesbian partner when she was in her early twenties. They planned and conceived the child as a couple. But Julie's partner left her for a man when the boy was only two and a half. Since the partner was the birth mother and they hadn't had any legal agreement, Julie's son was taken from her. She has remained in touch with him, but the birth mother called all the shots and kept them apart, especially in the years right after the breakup. Julie felt the loss of her son and her parenthood keenly, and her son felt and resented the loss of his other parent. Since then, Julie always wanted a child she could really call her own.

As Julie approached forty, she started thinking about single motherhood. "I'd been single so long, I'd kind of given up hope for someone to coparent with, and the clock was ticking." But Julie realized she didn't want just a donor, she wanted an involved dad. "Because I had that prior experience of parenting with a partner," Julie says, "I had an idea of how much work and exhaustion it could be to parent and work full-time. I know myself. I'm a so-cial person. I knew it would be a big priority for me to have a social life, or I wouldn't be as good as a mother. But as a single mom, how could I have a life outside of the baby? How would I find time to meet someone as a single parent? I didn't have family—my parents live in rural Canada—and at the time I didn't even have any friends with kids. I was so scared to be isolated and all alone with a child. That dovetailed with my natural inclination to have a known donor. I saw it as a real asset not only to me, but to the child, to have an involved coparent. I was thinking bigger—what if something happened to me? I was also wanting an extended family. I wanted the child to be part of a larger tribe. And I was worried about being solely financially responsible. I'm totally self-made," she says. Julie's parents are retired farm-ers and not in a position to contribute.

Julie met Paul, a gay man, through friends, and it turned out he wanted kids, too. He looked like a good catch as a donor. He had a stable job, a ca-reer as a lawyer, he was smart and well educated. They started to "date" each other, getting to know each other and talking about having a baby. "It was pretty informal. We didn't say we'd get together once a week, but it turned out that way. We did a lot of cultural events, like plays and movies. A lot of times other friends would come along. It wasn't that we were talking about babies every week." But over the course of two years, Julie and Paul really got to know a lot about each other and even met each other's family mem-bers. They talked about values and family. They discussed their careers, and where their careers might take them geographically. They shared their ideas on education and religion, as well as general issues about discipline. "We probably avoided talking about real-life scenarios and complications, be-cause we didn't want to scare the other off," Julie admits, in retrospect. "Like, how we'd spend holiday times, or how would you feel if I took him away at this age or that age." They hammered out an agreement in which they'd live in the same city until the child went to college. Though the agreement was somewhat flexible—it would be OK for one person to leave for a one- to two-year period, but the child would stay with the other parent, "I made the agreement with the understanding that I'd never be the one to leave," Julie says.

There was one sticking point with Julie: Paul wanted the child to reside with him half the time. "I never thought of it as a fifty-fifty thing," says Julie. "I always thought of myself as the custodial parent." But finally Julie agreed, an eye on her biological clock. "I was afraid he'd walk away, and I didn't have any other contenders."

Paul and Julie went ahead and made a baby, a little boy named Milo. From the beginning, the agreement has been both a blessing and a challenge. Paul was present at the birth—an unmedicated delivery in a natural birthing center—and since he was neither a partner nor exactly a close friend, it felt awkward. "I didn't want to lean on him literally or emotionally. I just sort of blocked him out. But I knew how much it meant to him." Then Julie had not anticipated how she would feel about sharing her infant son after her earlier parenting experience. It was like her baby was being taken away all over again. "When Milo wasn't with me, I missed him like I was missing an arm," Julie says flatly. "It's not like I worried that his father wasn't taking care of him, or didn't love him as much as I do, or that he wasn't happy," Julie says. Still, it was very hard on her. At about three months old, Paul took Milo to his apartment for an overnight. "I was so upset and distraught," Julie recalls. Additionally, she had not anticipated that having a child with Paul meant having a lifelong relationship with him. Her practical administrator's mind had jumped right over the emotional component to coparenting. "I thought of it as a business arrangement where we had an equal stake in the child," Julie says. "I think he thought of it more as a family." They hadn't really talked about that. Oops.

Though the arrangement has been quite difficult at times, "really there are a lot of benefits," Julie admits. "Just in terms of moral support, having someone to bounce ideas off of. I do like it that Milo knows he has this whole extended family all over D.C. and New England." And having a built-in babysitter has been great for Julie's social life. She's been able to date a lot, and has had two major relationships since her son was born. She and her current girlfriend have moved in together and are talking about being life partners. But that's where it gets sticky again: Julie already has a parenting partner—Paul.

"In terms of getting involved in a relationship, the parenting agreement has presented challenges I hadn't thought about," Julie admits. "My partner is not just having a relationship with me, she's having a relationship with my coparent." The three-way relationship involves three different schedules, feelings, and personalities. For example, sometimes Paul wants to juggle weekends around so he can go on a date. Julie wants to support Paul in his dating, but her girlfriend gets annoyed at changes in their plans. Also, Julie's girlfriend has taken over some parental responsibilities—she sets limits and disciplines Milo, in addition to having fun with him. But, as Julie points out, "she's not the same as Paul; she's not legally responsible for him, she doesn't take him to the doctor or to the dentist. It's an issue for her because she doesn't know how she fits in.

"If in time she feels more comfortable, she'll be more likely to step in as a real parent," Julie says. "But it would be easier for her if it had been a non-involved donor or a sperm-bank donor."

All in all, it's been a positive experience and Milo is thriving. But Julie's not certain she'd do it all over again the same way. "In retrospect," she says, "if I were independently wealthy, I would have done it on my own. I could have bought services, found male role models."

## GOOD THINGS COME IN THREES

Some single women end up providing their kids with even more than the standard number of parents. Catherine is on a mission to do just that. She and her best friend Joe were out dancing one night when Joe, a gay man with a long-term partner, said, "You know what would be really nice? I want to have a family, and I think you should be the one we do it with."

"I thought, Are you kidding?" remembers Catherine, who works in Manhattan and lives in New Jersey. But she thought Joe would be a really great father, and "the older I got, the more it became clear I wasn't going to have a family in the more orthodox way. The closer we got, the more logical it seemed." Catherine got to know Joe's partner, Kaysel, and the three of them talked about children. As different as they were—Joe, a white-bread native of Cape Cod; Kaysel, a Dominican immigrant with a born-again Christian mother; and Catherine, the first-generation daughter of conservative Eastern European immigrants—they came together on all child-rearing matters. "Even if we talked about religion or discipline or schooling, we all seemed to agree." Catherine bought a home three blocks from where Joe and Kaysel lived, and they started the process in earnest.

"It didn't actually get more complicated with three people," Catherine says. "In many ways it got easier. Having three people balanced everything out. There's always another person saying, well, I'll pick up that slack. And it helped make it easier for me to think about having a child. It became less overwhelming, and it helped me a lot in terms of how I can have this child and still get a lot done. It's nice because we have three incomes to contribute to this child's life."

One major issue was where the child would live. "I am the mom," Catherine told the two men. "I would love the child to live with me." Joe and Kaysel agreed that was the primary bond, but they all agreed that when the child got older, they could perhaps divide the time.

Then there was a small glitch over religion. "It was important to Kaysel and me that the child be baptized," Catherine says. "Joe said he didn't want to be part of it, but you guys can go do it. We keep coming up with compromises.

"I thought this was a pretty unorthodox situation," Catherine remembers. Turns out, not so much. At least, not in the big city. They mentioned the idea to their primary-care doctor, and it turned out that he had a couple of friends who had already done the same thing.

The more they talked, the better the coparenting idea sounded. Joe is a dance instructor who works afternoons and evenings. Catherine's job as a fashion designer means she has "a pretty erratic life. The hours are really horrible, and that's going to be the biggest challenge." And Kaysel is a vice president at a major bank. "He works like crazy, but he's just twenty minutes from home." Their schedules overlap, so there's barely any need for professional child care. Their personalities complement each other, too, Catherine feels. And while their various families may have trouble with the arrangement at first, Catherine thinks they'll come around, and in addition to a mom and two dads, there will be an incredibly rich extended family for the lucky child. "There will be a balance for this kid to thrive on—or be to-tally screwed up by!"

How will coparenting a child with her best friends affect her future love life? "Well," Catherine says sheepishly, "I don't know that there's anyone out there who wants to take something like this on. In many ways, emotionally, I don't feel like I need too many things, which doesn't exactly get me out the door. But there's one need Joe and Kaysel can't deal with, so . . . I should just go online and find somebody, just for fun."

Mikki Morrissette does Catherine one better. She has three daddies for her kids. "I'm really in favor of the coparenting and collaborative parenting thing," she says. Aware of the pain adopted kids can go through because they don't know their biological origin, Mikki used a friend as a donor for both of her kids. The donor is somewhat involved, though he is not able to be a reliable part of her kids' lives, so she has limited his contact with them so that her kids aren't put in the position of expecting more of a relationship than he can give. In addition to the donor, there's Mikki's ex-husband, who she remained good friends with. Seven years after their divorce, she had her first child as a single mom, and since then her ex has been a big part of the kids' lives. And ever since she remarried, her kids have her new husband, too, to go sledding with them and do other dad-type things.

Mikki's daughter was seven and a half when her mother and I spoke. "When she was five or six, she used to say she had three daddies: Real Daddy, Pretend Daddy, and Stepdaddy. Now she doesn't use those labels—she just calls them by their first names." But she still has the three daddies, three men who are special in her life, and for whom she is special, too.

# Coming Out About
# Single Motherhood

At a kid-friendly New Year's Eve party, keeping an eye on six-month-old Scott as he rolled around on the floor, I spoke to Mary, the single mom by choice of a four-year-old boy in New York City. At one point I asked what she told people when they asked about her son's father. She didn't have a ready answer. "I'm still not really comfortable with that," she admitted, glancing guiltily over at her son who, with the hostess's four-year-old, was gleefully cranking the salad spinner so it sounded more like a jet engine. "I'm going to have to deal with that before he picks up on my issues with it."

Mary's right, I think—if you feel ashamed or uncomfortable about your choice, that's going to have a negative effect on your child and his self-esteem. It's also likely that when people around you pick up on your discomfort, they'll take their cue from you and be less accepting than they might otherwise have been.

It's really a lot like coming out. Your desire for a child may be totally traditional, but as a single mom by choice, suddenly you're living an alternative lifestyle—especially if you used an anonymous donor. But for most single moms by choice, who are heterosexual and otherwise mainstream, it's hard to adjust to being considered "alternative," especially if what you'd been aiming for was a *Leave It to Beaver* kind of normalcy. And "coming out" isn't always so easy. I think I've gotten pretty comfortable coming out as gay, after a mere twenty-four years of practice. Even so, sometimes it's hard. Who wants to be the weirdo, right? (Well, some do, but I'm guessing most don't.) Being out as a lesbian makes it easier for me to embrace this other alternative label, "single mom by choice," but still I don't quite know how to respond when people ask me, "So, where's Scott's dad?"

I've tried out a breezy "Oh, Scott's a sperm-donor baby." It sounds OK in my head, but when it comes out of my mouth it seems slightly disrespectful of Scott, and the word "sperm" sounds a touch shocking, since it's not normally used in casual social interactions. I have tried "His dad? He's donor number 555" (not the real number), which had a funny ring to it in my mind, but not in real conversation. I think I have settled on a simple "Scott doesn't have a dad; I had him on my own." It lets folks know the unusual answer in a gentler way. Then if they want to know more, I can go into the donor story.

I spoke to Melissa when her twin boys were just eleven weeks old, and she'd been trying out a few things, too. When she walked out of the hospital after the birth with her mom and uncle, the security guard asked, "Where's the father?"

"I turned around and said, 'Denmark,' point blank, and walked away," Melissa says. (She used a Danish sperm bank.)

She's come up with another glib answer: "I gave up on Mr. Right and went for Mr. Petri Dish," she tells people who ask. She says she gets funny looks, as if she is being shockingly irreverent about her sons' origins. Those people need to get a life, she feels. "Not everyone realizes the seriousness of the thought and the effort it took to take me to this conclusion."

One thing is guaranteed: If you become a single mom, people *will* ask about the father. "I can't tell you how many times, when I say I have a baby, people say, 'Oh, what does your husband do?' " says Erron.

Alice, the telecommunications executive from Maryland, recalls her first foray into coming out as a single mom by donor insemination. "When I told my boss, he said, 'Congratulations! I didn't know you were seeing anyone. What's the father's role?' " says Alice.

"The father is a number," Alice replied, then felt a little weird about her own answer. "I wasn't prepared for it," she says now. "It was the first time." Now, what she tells people depends a little on who's asking. "A lot of times

I'll just say I'm a single mother and the father's not involved," she says. Saying that makes Alice, who is Black, appear to represent a racial stereotype she isn't particularly comfortable with, but it also discourages further questions. "But if it's a single woman in her thirties," Alice says, "I'll say I went to the bank and took out a deposit."

"Most everybody knows I'm a single parent," says Debrah. "I don't lie about it." But she feels no need to tell the entire story to everyone. "When people say, 'Does he look like his father?' if I don't know them well, I just say no." When she enrolled her son in preschool, which she has done at two different schools, she has been asked if there's anything special the school should know. "I say he doesn't have a father, he has an anonymous sperm donor." It's been a nonissue for Debrah. "The school, they just want to make sure the child's OK."

"I do get a lot of honest questions," says Cheri. "Like, about the donor: Does he know about Jack? I've become a lot more comfortable with talking about it." Cheri feels that being open and telling the truth is essential. "I don't want Jack to ever feel ashamed or think I'm ashamed of the way he was conceived."

When Elisa was pregnant, she says, "I was on a mission to educate the world." So to set people straight when they assumed she had a husband, she answered every question and volunteered her single-mom-by-choice status even when no one asked. "I didn't want anyone to have anything to gossip about," she says. What she found was an unexpected group of cheerleaders—older women, ages fifty to eighty-five, who were married with kids. "They'd say, 'Oh, that's the way to do it; if I had had the chance to do it that way, I would have!' "

For Tauz, who is four months pregnant and lives on a Native American reservation near Santa Fe, single motherhood isn't the big social hurdle; it's donor insemination. (I spoke to at least one white woman from a rural area who said the same thing.) "There's a lot of single moms here, not by choice," Tauz says. That's not a big surprise for anyone. But artificial insemination is something else. "People are surprised, shocked that I would do that; have a child with a total stranger. Nobody in this pueblo has ever done that." She hasn't announced it to the whole pueblo, but she does tell people one by one. "There's lots of questions and a lot of curiosity about it," she says. "I tell people because I'm a lesbian and I don't want them to think I just shacked up with someone." Genealogy is very important within her tribe's culture, so anonymous-donor insemination is potentially an issue in that respect as well. Even though she picked someone who's part Native American, "I won't know the native blood of the donor [i.e., which tribe he's from]," she admits. Tauz says that even though her dad is African-American and Native American, people on the reservation never really accepted him as Native American because his tribe was not native to New Mexico. But she feels that despite his or her unusual roots, her child will be more accepted than her father was. "When they're born here and they're raised here and they participate in the dances from a very young age, there's more acceptance."

Carol, who has three kids, also had more reactions to her method of conception than to her single motherhood. Carol adopted her first child from Africa as a single mom. Her next child was born within her eight-year marriage to a man she later divorced, and the third was conceived through in vitro fertilization as a single mom again. Both times she chose single motherhood, she says, "I didn't get any of the 'single parent—wow!' type of reaction." She explains that's because single motherhood, through adoption or through not-so-accidental pregnancy, is pretty common in the Black community. "For a thousand and one reasons, there's a limited pool of eligible Black men," she says, mentioning the high rate of Black men in prison and other factors. "It's a darn shame, but as a result, you wind up with a lot of nice, bright, educated African-American women who are single and want families." Many of them make it happen. What's not so common is using artificial insemination or in vitro fertilization, the method Carol chose. No one in her community had ever heard of anyone who'd done it.

"I'd say IVF and their jaws would hang open. Then I'd say in vitro fertilization. That wouldn't help at all. The jaws would still be hanging open. Then I'd say test-tube babies."

"So, it's sort of like sleeping with someone you don't know," they'd say.

"No, it's not at all like that!" Carol would reply.

"Well, if you had told me, I could have found someone for you."

It simply was not computing. "No, I wanted it this way," Carol would say, explaining that she didn't want to pressure or trick some guy into being a father.

After the initial shock, she said, people she knew were kind of excited to know someone who'd done something they'd only ever heard about on TV.

"Wow, that is bizarre!" they'd say. "Well, what if he has a hundred other kids?"

"Great!" Carol would reply. "Then if my son gets sick there'll be so many other opportunities for a new kidney."

"Basically, they thought I was insane," Carol says, "but they loved me and wished me well." In fact, her church has been incredibly supportive. Her minister has a usual spiel in which he lists different ways that children have come into his parishioners' lives, "whether by traditional marriage or adoption or step-parenting. . . ." After Carol had her third child, she says, "He started throwing in in vitro fertilization, and I was like, 'That's so sweet!' " So now, when the subject of children comes up, the minister will say, "whether by in vitro fertilization," Carol reports, "and the whole church turns and smiles at me."

## KEEPING QUIET ABOUT THE DETAILS OF YOUR CHILD'S CONCEPTION

Not all single moms are totally open about how their families were created. When strangers or acquaintances ask Samantha about her daughter's dad, "I'll say, 'The father's not involved.' There'll be a look, she adds, but then people generally don't pursue it. "I feel like it is her story, not mine," Samantha explains. "If I tell people now, they'll always know." At the same time, Samantha says, "I'd like my daughter to know the truth at an early enough age, and to know that it's not weird."

Yet when Samantha *has* been open with people, she has gotten a warm reception. "I think in a lot of ways there's less of a stigma [with choosing single motherhood] than with an accidental pregnancy," she says. When she told a couple of older, conservative people, she was surprised to find that they really respected her for what she did. "It's the virgin birth," Samantha guesses, as a way of explaining the unexpected support from conservative friends. "I think there's also a lot of respect because it was a choice."

Though Elisa was open about how she became pregnant, she became more private about the issue once her daughter Skye was born, feeling that it was Skye's story now, and no longer Elisa's place to share it so openly. "She's going to be friends with kids at school, and maybe she doesn't want them to know." Her teachers will know, but Elisa no longer feels OK about being as open about how her daughter was conceived as she was when she was pregnant.

"I think a lot of people don't want to ask questions," says Suzie, who has two daughters as a single mom. But "people look at you like, 'Um, are you going to explain?'" Usually, Suzie doesn't. "If somebody got divorced, I don't think they'd go into detail about their personal life." But by saying nothing, Suzie allows people to come up with their own stories, which may be pretty far from her family's reality. When people do know, she finds them "supportive but curious."

Putting an end to people coming up with their own inaccurate explanations is one reason why Charlene sometimes tells acquaintances or strangers the details of her daughter's conception. "Eventually you tell them the truth because you don't want them to think there's baby-daddy drama or something," she says. But the questions rankle her. "I don't want to have to explain myself," she says. "That's not their business. I don't tell you I have my period if you're a stranger on the street."

Charlene's not alone in feeling that her daughter's sperm-bank origin is socially on par with discussing body functions. Many single moms feel it's a highly private matter, probably because of the sex-related words they have to use to talk about it—"sperm" and "insemination." In reality, telling someone you had your child through anonymous-donor insemination is not any more intimate than telling them that you're married to your kid's dad. If you tell them the latter, you're basically letting them into your sex life, saying, "My husband got an erection, slid his penis into my vagina, and ejaculated; that's how we got our kid." But of course, it's so common that no one's mind goes straight to the details in that way.

The "ick" factor of choosing single motherhood is similar to the way being gay is sexualized in people's minds. If you mention you have a husband, people think of it as a social relationship, not a sexual one. But tell someone you have a same-sex partner, and suddenly you're flaunting your sexuality in everyone's face. Similarly, if you used an anonymous donor, even if you don't throw the word "sperm" in there, that's what some people will think about. I think the only way to get past it is to take a deep breath, be open about it, and wait for society to catch up. In my opinion, shame and secrecy will only breed more problems. And let's get real: All of us started with sperm.

## WHY DISCLOSURE MATTERS

Why do we even need to tell people anything? Because they ask, and it's a perfectly normal question, in my opinion. And because I feel it's important to live one's life openly and honestly. More importantly, what message would it send to my son if I tried to hide his origins? It would suggest to him, and to everyone, that it's something to be ashamed of. So even though it might be a little uncomfortable for me at first, I think coming out is important. Words like "donor" sound weird because they're new. We're not used to wrapping our mouths, or our minds, around them. But the more they are used, the less strange they'll seem to us and to everyone around us, and that's crucial for our kids. That's my opinion, but the experts I interviewed who work with donor-conceived children agree.

Wendy Kramer of the Donor Sibling Registry talks to donor-conceived children every day, and she says that secrecy around donor insemination can be damaging. "Secrecy implies shame," she says. "Oh, it's a secret?" kids ask. "Why is it a secret?" The answer kids often come up with is that there's something wrong with the way they were made, she says. "The more you apply secrecy, the more it implies shame, and I think that's what kids get if their parents maintain secrecy. I tell people as much as I can: Don't do that."

In Wendy's family, donor insemination was not a secret, and she says that as a result, her son's attitude was, "I'm a donor kid—so?" He felt fine about it because that's the message he was getting at home, and "no one's ever called him on it," Wendy says. "There's no secrecy, there's no shame, there's no 'Oh, this is something we tell some people and not other people.' "

Diane Ehrensaft, a psychologist who has worked with many families who have used donor insemination, wholeheartedly supports parents' impulses to protect their kids and maintain privacy. But is privacy what's really at issue? Dr. Ehrensaft suggests weighing your desire for privacy against "inadvertently giving a message of shame to your child." Examine your desire for privacy, she suggests. If you find that the root of it is that you feel bad about how you got pregnant, it's important to work through that by finding a support group, where you can see how others have dealt with these feelings, or going for short-term counseling. "For your child's sake, it's important to address those anxieties so that you're not burdened with them and so you don't pass them to your child inadvertently," Dr. Ehrensaft says. "As with most things in raising children, whenever there are issues, your kids will do as well as you do." She says there are some "exceptional circumstances" where it may be best not to disclose—for example, if your child is mentally handicapped and could not absorb the information properly—but that openness is generally the healthier policy. But how to say it, exactly? Dr. Ehrensaft offers some ideas. "We're a one-parent family," she suggests. You could just leave it at that, or say, "It's me and Timmy, there is no dad. We used a sperm donor." If "sperm" sounds too graphic to you, you can say "artificial insemination," or, to get even further away from embarrassing fluids, "assisted reproductive technology."

As uncomfortable as it can be to discuss alternative conception in specific terms, it can be necessary for clarity's sake, in part because people are so unfamiliar with the concept. Marcy finds she has to say, " 'artificial insemination,' because if I just say 'insemination,' people think that's slang for 'some guy who wasn't worth very much who I just slept with one night.' "

When you speak about your choice of donor insemination to your child or to others, "the more it's a tale full of pride, the more the child will feel proud," says Dr. Ehrensaft. Conversely, "the more it's a tale of woe, the more the child will think there's something wrong with his conception." She recommends parents tell their child the story in simple language very early on, before the child is really old enough to understand it. That way "you get to practice, for one thing," she says. If you are low-key about it and have a positive tone of voice, that will say more to your child than even the words themselves.

Kids may run across challenges on the playground at some point, and moms can help them by letting them know "it's the other kids' problem, not theirs," Dr. Ehrensaft says. But the strongest defense is the feeling of pride you can help your kid internalize. If you are anticipating any issues, you can tell your child, "We're really proud of the family we have, and some people don't understand that, so we have to teach them." That's if the issue is a mild and transitory one, which it's likely to be. Based on the experiences of the women I have interviewed, choosing single motherhood and conceiving through donor insemination is pretty well accepted in most of this country. "I think there's been a sea change," Dr. Ehrensaft says. But some communities may be more accepting than others. "If your child is in a really hostile environment and you have the opportunity to change that, that's better than trying to 'toughen up' your child," Dr. Ehrensaft cautions.

Openness and honesty about donor insemination can be important on a personal level for you and your child for the reasons Wendy Kramer and Diane Ehrensaft cited above. But I'd argue that coming out about choosing single motherhood is also important politically, for the same reason that coming out is a political imperative within the gay community. People with openly gay friends, family members, and acquaintances are a lot less eager to discriminate against gays as a group. It's the same with women who have chosen to be single mothers. Mark Davis, the columnist and radio talkshow host, wrote in a 2007 column that any reasons for choosing single motherhood amount to "selfish twaddle," and opined that single moms are "bringing kids into the world with the express intent of denying them a married mother and father." (I love that! We diabolical single moms go to all these lengths to have kids because we want to *deny them things*!) Do you suppose Mark would have written this if he'd actually gotten to know a single mom by choice? Unlikely. Now, Mark's opinions are fine for Mark to have. It's a free country. But put enough Marks together and they have the potential to get lawmakers thinking they need to pass laws that punish single moms and make life harder for their kids. That's why those of us living "alternative" lifestyles need to be open and upbeat about it, because otherwise we may find ourselves the dehumanized scapegoat of someone else's ill-informed political or religious diatribe.

Of course, that doesn't mean every stranger needs to know every detail—there are many times when the full story is overkill. When someone asks me if Scott's father is tall, for example, I simply say yes, and leave it at that.

## CONFRONTING SINGLE-MOM STEREOTYPES

One barrier to coming out as a single mom by choice is the fear of having to take on stereotypes. For example, the idea that if you choose to have a baby without a man, that must mean you're a lesbian. As a bona-fide lesbian, I had no idea that stereotype was out there—I knew that the overwhelming majority of single moms by choice are straight. I assumed that, if anything, lesbian single moms like me were an invisible minority. But a handful of the straight single moms I spoke to have had people wonder about their sexual orientation.

"Coming out as straight is interesting," says Kristen, who is heterosexual and trying to conceive as a single mom. She told her doctor she was single and was asked before a procedure, "Do you want to bring your partner?" The doctor was assuming that "single" actually meant "in a lesbian relationship." The same thing happened when she accompanied a pregnant single-mom-by-choice friend to the hospital when she started bleeding. "We were treated as lesbian partners." Kristen's philosophically glad that there's acceptance of diversity from the health-care professionals in New York, but she finds being taken for gay a little uncomfortable and irritating.

Charlene has gotten the "Are you gay?" question, too, but that's nothing compared to having people assume she's "that single mom on welfare," which she says happens all the time because she's African-American. It's been a real shock. "I've become that stereotype, and that's a Black person I don't know." Charlene had an upper-middle-class upbringing in Birmingham, Alabama. Her dad was a doctor. People in her set went to Harvard, Princeton, Fisk, and Howard. Her parents were married fifty years before her dad died. "*The Cosby Show,* that was my family," she says. "The last thing we were going to do is be unwed mothers. That was something poor Black people did. To bring that stigma on my daughter, that's hard for me." Still, she feels it's important for educated single Black women to know that choosing single motherhood is an option for them. A lot of older successful Black women Charlene knows didn't have children and have regrets about it. And Charlene says that when she sees women of color coming to Single Mothers by Choice meetings, they come in about five years later than the white women, with the result that their childbearing dreams may be less likely to come true. "They come in at, like, forty-eight, and I'm like, damn, that's way too late." Charlene has heard people within the community say, "I didn't know Black folks did that." Her answer: "We *do* do this. And you need to know that you have a choice."

Still, for an educated woman of color who has paid big bucks to a sperm bank and a doctor, being stereotyped this way is annoying to say the least. "One of my clients asked, 'Weren't you careful?'" says Tauz, who is African-American and Native American. "Yeah, I was really careful," she replied. "As a matter of fact, I paid for it."

Melle has a Ph.D.—and three kids as a single mom by choice. But because she's Black and has dreadlocks, she says, she gets comments like, "You're not married, right?"

"Single mom by choice is such a minority, when they see me the 'by choice' thing is irrelevant," she says.

It's a double-edged sword, though, these women say, because the fact that they apparently fit a stereotype also means they get fewer questions. In Melle's experience, "out in the world in general, people are not surprised" to see a Black single mother. The other Black women I spoke to all said that although they are uncomfortable with the stereotype that doesn't fit them, there was a certain benefit to *not* being perceived as an oddity. "Being African-American makes it harder and easier," says Alice. "There are so many single mothers, so nobody flinches."

"It lets you be part of a club," says Charlene. "It's assumed you're struggling like everyone else." It's a club Charlene, with her privileged background, wasn't part of. "I didn't think of myself as a Black woman in this process," she says. "But all of a sudden, once I had my child, I became a 'real' Black woman."

In addition to forcing you to confront stereotypes regarding sexual orientation and race, single motherhood can stereotype you politically. Jennifer is one of the women I spoke to who identifies as conservative, and she's quite irritated that her decision to become a single mom is seen as a "liberal" one. "I see my decision as being completely aligned with my conservative beliefs," Jennifer says. "Conservatives are most highly concerned with personal responsibility, versus liberals who care more for group rights. I am not having a baby because it's my right to do so, but because I have worked hard to be in a position where I can bring a child into the world and take full responsibility for him or her. I am highly educated and financially independent; I can be sure that I will have the time, money, and interest to raise a child as well as, if not better than, most of the children I see growing up in my city. I will take my child to church; I will raise my child to think about how he or she can really make the world a better place. I will not ask for social assistance or send my child to a fancy private school if it means I have to ask someone else to pay for it. I will treat my child as a wonderful gift as well as a lifelong responsibility. And what could be more conservative than that?"

One Sunday the first summer of my son's life, when he was maybe five weeks old, my mom and her favorite golf buddy—let's call her Mrs. Smith—had signed up to host their church's after-service coffee hour. This was pretty funny, as neither my mom nor Mrs. Smith is the coffee-hour-hostess type, not even remotely. They are both dry wits more at home on the golf course than in the kitchen. I can't speak for Mrs. Smith, but my mom would much rather shovel manure or wash a dog that's been sprayed by a skunk than throw a party. I'm the opposite, so while the chocolate-chip cookies were baking I set Scott in his bouncy seat and started making a carved basket out of a watermelon and filling it with little balls of pink, orange, and green. Then we loaded cookies, melon basket, and baby into the station wagon and headed for the Church on the Cape.

Anyhow, Mrs. Smith is a laid-back yet proper New Englander who speaks with perhaps a touch of an upper-class lockjaw, like Katharine Hepburn. She also happens to be very close to that local über-Republican family, the Bushes. After I set the melon out on the folding table in the coffee-hour room and she set out her store-bought cheese and crackers and coffee cake, Mrs. Smith and I started to chat, me holding Scott in a sling.

"So, Louise, where's your husband?" she asked conversationally, in that somewhat brusque, intimidating, Hepburn sort of way.

I took a deep breath and gave her my usual spiel. "Oh, Scott's a sperm-donor baby," I said, attempting a fast-talking upbeat breeziness. "I always wanted children and I didn't have a partner and my clock was ticking, so . . ."

Mrs. Smith seemed fascinated, and quizzed me on some of the details of this newfangled way to make a baby.

Later, my mom reported, Mrs. Smith cornered her in the church kitchen.

"I think it's just wonderful that Louise has the baby," she told my mom. Then she added: "*And I know how she got him!*"

This from a proper older woman, a conservative old-school Republican. And, not that we can be held responsible for those around us, but this woman is close to the guy who thinks someone like me getting married is such a threat to our nation that he proposed a constitutional amendment to prevent it! It's amazing how thoughts like that can lose their urgency when one gets to know the "other," whether it be the gay couple or the single mom, and can see them as the human beings that they are.

Mikki Morrissette has found that to be true in most cases she's observed. "Once people see choice motherhood in action, a lot of the prejudices fall by the wayside, unless they come from a deeply conservative political or religious place."

Sadly, single motherhood is only an unusual thing when you have an infant or toddler. Many of the moms I talked to said the same thing Marcy does: "As my son gets older, more and more people just assume I got a divorce."

## NOT TELLING WHILE INSEMINATING

Some women choose not to tell until it's too late for anyone to have an opinion about it. This can be wise in some cases—people warm much more quickly to a real child than to the idea of choosing single motherhood. But sometimes the fear of judgment is unfounded. Michele was terrified of disapproval when, after her divorce, she had an accidental pregnancy with a casual new boyfriend and decided to keep the child. That pregnancy ended in miscarriage, but she learned, to her surprise, that her friends and family were "ecstatic" for her to have a child. They did not have a problem with her being a single mom—their biggest worry was that the divorce meant that she might not be able to be a mom at all. So when she started to try to conceive through artificial insemination, her fears were gone and she shared with everyone. "I talk to my father about it," she says. "I talk to everybody and anybody about it. Everyone knows what's going on."

Catherine, who's trying to get pregnant and plans to coparent with her gay best friends, has chosen not to share the news with her conservative parents. "I think I'm in for a bit of a battle," she says. "I know they're not going to be jumping and shouting from the rooftops." Catherine, who is white, was engaged to a Black man at one point. When she told her mom about her wedding plans, the reaction was, "I hope you're not serious. As your mother I would do anything to stop you from throwing your life away." Needless to say, Catherine is not eager to hear a similar reaction to her childbearing plan. "I'm not without hope," Catherine says, "but I have to be realistic. They could very well turn around and cut themselves off from me and I have to be ready for that."

"I haven't told my father," says Min, who's trying to conceive as well. "I just don't want any additional stress. I know he'll be afraid for me." But does she anticipate a problem? "I don't think he'll be surprised, really," Min adds. "Once it settles in, I think he'll be supportive."

Min has told friends, and says the one friend who was initially not supportive—feeling that a child should have two parents—finally came around. "I have a group of aunties assembled," she says. "Are they going to help me raise the child? Probably not," Min admits. "But I'm counting on them for moral support."

Nicole, who's thirty-six and trying to conceive with anonymous-donor sperm, hasn't gotten a lot of bad reactions. "People have been very surprised, but then very happy." Her mom was thrilled—"She just wants to have a grandchild," Nicole says. "One of my brothers isn't so much against my single-motherhood plans," Nicole reports, "but he plugs his ears and sings 'La la la' at the top of his lungs at any mention of 'sperm donor,' and, yes, he's thirty." Her other brother did take issue with it, however. "I cannot agree with your project. I think you're selling yourself short," he told her. "There are more natural, more conventional ways to do this. And you are planning to deprive a child of any connection to one of the most important people in his life—which may leave him feeling more empty and alone than you are feeling right now." And she "got into it" with her cousin's husband, a man from a very traditional Italian family.

Nicole was visiting. "He's sitting in his nice house, holding his new baby and his other child, and says to me, 'So, when are you going to take matters into your own hands?' " He was referring to marriage and family. "Well, actually," Nicole replied, "I've made a decision to have a baby on my own."

"He flew at me," Nicole recalls. " 'You can't have a child,' he told me. 'Do you know how hard this is? Do you *know* how hard this is? You live in an apartment, you don't have a husband. It's not fair to the child.' " Nicole was furious. "Making up my mind to do this was a very emotional process." She did not appreciate the judgment, especially coming from someone who, she felt, had had everything handed to him on a silver platter by his wealthy parents. "I know I can do this," she told him. "I haven't had everything given to me. I'm the most resourceful person I know. I can do this." The idea that it's unfair to the kids makes her angry. "I think there's a lot of stuff in life that's not fair to kids. I think it would be better for a child to have a father, but at the same time, there are a lot of bad fathers out there. Just because the father's in the picture doesn't mean it will be better for the child.

"People are happy for me, and that's exciting," Nicole says. She comes from a rural area that's conservative and traditional. But, she adds, "The flip side of being from a small rural place is that there are a lot of single moms out there. When I tell people my plans, they're more shocked by the process than the outcome. The fact that I'm going to a sperm bank has got everyone giggling and laughing." Nicole isn't too worried about the gossip. "People will definitely talk, and that's fine. Because the next time something comes up to talk about, they'll talk about that, too."

## TELLING FAMILY

When I was three and a half months pregnant, I sent out an e-mail to my whole extended family—about eighty names. Ostensibly, this was to tell them about my new e-mail address and Web site (oh, and by the way I'm single and happily pregnant). In reality, it was my way of letting them all know the deal without my mother's having to go through the embarrassment of doing it with them one by one.

I was delighted to get nothing but positive responses. Just about the first e-mail I got back was from my ninety-one-year-old great-aunt Elizabeth, the matriarch and oldest living member of my conservative Southern Republican family, whose last missive to the family was taking all eighty-some of us gracefully but firmly to task for not writing thank-you notes. I am sure she was beyond shocked by my choice. But that's not the message she sent me.

"Congratulations!" she e-mailed. (E-mailed! At ninety-one!) "What a brave thing to do."

After hearing "brave" a few too many times, I have decided that it's a code word for "weird," but still.

Who knows what's being said behind my back, but to my face all I've gotten is kindness and support, and even baby gifts.

Like me, most women I spoke to were surprised at the positive reception they had. "I thought they were going to give me hell," says Jocelyn. "My parents have historically had the attitude of 'Don't do anything that would embarrass us,' or that their friends' children wouldn't do it." Jocelyn consulted her siblings about what their parents' reaction was likely to be. "Three out of three kids thought they would flip out." The actual reaction? "They were thrilled. Go figure!"

Grandparents in particular often turn out to be much more supportive than the single moms would have expected. "I told my grandmother I was pregnant, and how I got pregnant," Cheri remembers. "She was thrilled about the grandchild, but asked why I hadn't told her I was planning this. I said I was concerned about what she might think." Grandma's response? "I don't know how you got pregnant, but I'm not really sure how I got pregnant, either!" Another single mom's grandmother made her priorities clear: "I don't care whether you girls get married," she told Marcy, "I just want a great-grandchild!"

"I wasn't sure if my ninety-year-old grandfather would disown me," says Melissa. "But he's been great!"

"I got almost uniformly wonderful and warm responses," says Diana, who lives in a conservative Midwestern city. "A couple of men, both family friends in their sixties and seventies, were initially resistant to the idea—perhaps they just didn't know how to react—but it didn't take long for them to come around. In the context of knowing me and my family, they came to accept and welcome my children as everyone else I knew had. They have been incredibly supportive. One of them helped to lead my daughter's baby-naming ceremony. Interestingly, the other one has a daughter who, about a year after me, herself had a daughter through an anonymous donor."

Cheri had a great reaction from her parents, and her sister, though concerned for her, was supportive. But Cheri's mom's side of the family is Mormon and very conservative. One great-aunt in particular had a problem with what Cheri was doing: "She thought it was like cloning, it was really crazy." Cheri's mom responded in the fiercely supportive and protective way most people can only dream that their moms would do. "Mom sent a letter explaining what I was doing and what it meant to me and what it meant to them, and said she hoped [my aunt] could be supportive, but if she couldn't be, there would be no contact." The tough love worked. "My aunt called and said, 'We're in Idaho, these things don't really happen around here, give me a chance to get used to it.' " Sure enough, she got used to it, and there have been visits and gifts exchanged. In fact, one of the great-aunt's sons was asking Cheri about her single-motherhood experience on behalf of his daughter, who is twenty-eight and has PCOS, the same fertility challenge that Cheri has. "He said it would be sad if his daughter never had the chance to have children."

"At a family level, it can transcend politics," says Kristen, who was adopted as a toddler. Her mom's decision to adopt two Black kids as a single mom could have been an opportunity for judgment and rejection by her white Republican relatives, but that's not what happened at all. "My sister and I always felt valued by our family," recalls Kristen, who expects the same acceptance for her future child.

"At first, my parents were a little like [pronounced with exaggerated slowness], 'OK,' " says Jessica. "I think they were a little nervous because I didn't have a relationship, that I would have this child and dump a whole lot of emotional stuff on the child. And I think that's a valid concern. But they realized it wasn't about having a child to fulfill some need in me. It's a much different thing to want a child than to want to be a mother. I wanted to be a mother. I wanted the *job*."

Sometimes the parents of a single mom by choice realize that they even prefer it this way. "Before I gave birth to my first daughter, my parents went on a hospital tour for grandparents," says Ellen, who has had two kids as a single mom. "They explained my single-mother situation, and the other grandparents said, 'You're so lucky! There's no competing grandparents, no difficult son-in-law—just a direct line to the grandkids!' "

When Ellen's parents first found out she planned to be a single mom, they were thrilled. Her dad started out all politically correct and trying not to pressure her: "I think that's great, it's your body and you can do whatever you want." And then he instantly followed up with, "But if it's a boy you need to name him Frank. . . ." Ellen laughs both ruefully and appreciatively at his level of involvement and excitement.

Ellen's having a child as a single mom has made her family closer. "We're more involved as a family," she says. "I call my mom four or five times a day, about medical stuff, what to eat, I call in the morning to report on what happened the evening before, I call when I pick the kids up at day care to let them know how they are." Far from being any kind of disappointment, Ellen's single-mom decision has been a joy and a blessing to her parents. "I am glad that I was able to make my parents so happy."

When Marcy told her parents—she waited until she was ten weeks pregnant—her mom was supportive, her dad "a little bit more wary of it," she says. But she got the warmest reaction from her grandmother. "I don't care whether you girls get married," she said, "I just want a great-grandchild!"

The hardest part for Lisa S. was telling her daughter (from a previous marriage), who was ten at the time and knew nothing of her mom's plans. "I didn't want her to be part of all the ups and downs of trying to conceive," says Lisa. At first her daughter was shocked: " 'Mom, what did you do?!' " recalls Lisa. But then she was thrilled and teary: "Mom, you're having a baby!" Lisa's "very liberal" family was quite supportive, having helped her pick the donor. "My brother-in-law probably had the hardest time with it, because he's an Orthodox rabbi, but he hasn't said anything to me about it," Lisa says. "He certainly hasn't treated my son any differently from my daughter."

My family had known forever that I wanted kids, and they'd had nearly two decades to adjust to my being gay, and so the single-mom-artificial-insemination thing was not exactly a big shock. There was probably some mild discomfort, especially for my mom, but I think they were mostly just excited for me and looking forward to a new baby. So it was most awkward, and funniest, when I told my niece and nephew, then six and eight, that I was pregnant. (My littlest niece, Sydney, was only one and a half and so wasn't a big part of the conversation.) We were all in my sister's SUV, driving down to Virginia for Christmas, and I picked a point where they were starting to get really bored to give them the exciting news.

"But how?" Tyler asked. "You don't have a husband."

"That's right," I said, and explained how I really wanted a baby and wanted to have one before I was too old, so since I didn't have a husband, I went to a sperm bank. "Have you ever heard of a sperm bank?" I asked. He had—apparently my sister had gone over it a while back to prep him for my announcement. I spelled out the very simple version of sperm and egg making baby, which he was also familiar with, and about the nice man who gave his sperm so that other people can have babies. All that seemed fine. Then he asked, "But how does the man donate his sperm?"

"Well, he goes to the bank, and he makes the donation," I said.

"But exactly *how* does he make the donation?" Tyler asked.

"Well, it's a simple procedure that happens at the bank," I hedged.

"But *what exactly* happens?" Tyler persisted. "How do they get the sperm?"

At this point I looked at my sister and said, "You take it from here." She told him that he was too young to understand. I loved Tyler's logical answer, which he repeated a couple times before he gave up and moved on:

"Well, if I'm too young to understand it, then just tell me anyway, and it won't be a big deal because I won't understand it!"

Other than being irritated by that little unsolved mystery, my niece and nephew were thrilled, and they especially loved the nickname my friend Sally had given the baby: "Fluffy." The next morning the first words out of my niece's mouth were, "How's Fluffy?" and she asked me that just about every hour on the hour for the entire week.

Sometimes family reaction is a negative surprise. Suzie's parents and sister were quite supportive of her first pregnancy, with her ex-boyfriend as the known donor. Since it was the product of a relationship, in a way, they were able to understand it as the "accident" it was certainly not. They were not as supportive of her second pregnancy using an anonymous donor, despite the abuse and heartache that the known donor had caused both Suzie and her daughter. "With my sister it was more of a religious thing," Suzie explains. "She had a problem with me making a *decision* to be a single mom. It was one thing to have a child with someone and have it not work out. But it wasn't morally right to have a child without a father." The family has since come around, though. The arrival of the child tends to do that with all but the most hardened of hearts.

"My dad was mortified; my mom was ecstatic," recalls Nina, who used a gay friend as a known donor. "I think it's a control thing," Nina says of her dad. "He's a Lutheran bishop and he sort of believes I'm damaged and it's like adultery, even though we didn't have sex and we're not married. He's worried that I won't get married ever, that no one is going to want to take on this kind of baggage." On the plus side, Nina says, "This will be his only grandchild and he says he won't take it out on the child."

Nina has had a warm reception from most others. "Everybody at my church has been supportive," and she feels that, in a way, the trail was already blazed by other members of her congregation. There are three single women who have adopted from China, and at least a few married couples who have used reproductive technology. "I feel like this is the same thing," Nina says. "My pastor came and congratulated me and was supportive."

Since Nina has been an active member of her church, serving as youth group advisor until recently, the support for her pregnancy was a relief. She is sad that her father is disapproving, but she says she mostly feels sad for him: "He's taking some joy he could be feeling away from himself. And it is weird because he lives next door," Nina says. (They both live on a family farm outside the city with "nine chickens, a horse, a mule, and a few dogs.") "But he's going to baptize the baby, so . . ." Nina is hopeful that the arrival of the grandchild will smooth over some of her dad's objections.

Even though her dad hasn't been entirely supportive emotionally, Nina knows her family will be there for her when push comes to shove, and that's a big part of her support system, as it is for many single moms by choice. "My dad's next door, his sister is in another house, my cousin lives down by the barn. There's going to be someone who can watch my child for ten minutes while I run to the store."

"My mom was not happy," says Shannon, who waited to tell her parents until she was already a few months along. "She said it was a mistake, I was ruining my chances for a good life, I was limiting myself socially and career-wise." Her mom is doing better now, Shannon reports, but she is still not accepting. On the plus side, when little Rowena was born, she says, "My dad and stepmom were very supportive. In fact, my dad offered to come down and help." About a week after delivery, Shannon, who had no assistance at all, called him in tears, and he arrived as soon as he could. "Being from the 'Mom-does-it-all' generation, he didn't know quite what to do, but he was very sweet," she says. Though she now lives in the suburbs of Los Angeles, Shannon dreams of having a farm where she can grow "rows and rows of vegetables and fruit trees," and have a cow and chickens. Now, prompted by their excitement over their granddaughter, her dad and stepmom are building a guesthouse just for Shannon and Rowena on their farm in central Oregon. "My dream is close to coming true," says Shannon.

Erron had mixed results, too. "My dad comes from a wealthy Jewish family and they were embarrassed that I was pregnant out of wedlock," she says. But her mom has been supportive and helps with child care.

Sometimes loved ones are just concerned for your well-being. That's what Anne, who had one child with an ex-boyfriend, found when she shared her decision to have another baby as a single mom by choice. "When I announced this to my friends and family, they said, 'Why would you do this? Why would you ever take on this incredible amount of work by yourself?' " recalls Anne.

Parents also don't want their kids to be alone. "My dad asked me had I given up on men," says Charlene. "I said, 'If you introduce me to Mr. Not-So-Bad, I'll marry him tomorrow.' "

"I don't want you to give up," her father said in reply.

## TELLING PEOPLE AT WORK

When Suzie was pregnant with her second child as a single mom, her boss announced that she'd been promoted. Suzie went to him and let him know of her pregnancy.

"What are you talking about?" her boss asked, perplexed.

"I did a Murphy Brown," Suzie replied.

"Oh," he said. She got the promotion anyway.

Later, Suzie's boss said, "Well, we don't want to ask any questions, but we just assume you're a lesbian."

"As long as you get the job done, he doesn't care who you are," Suzie says. But how does she feel being pegged as a lesbian when she is not? "It's fine, I just laugh about it."

"In the military, you don't have the luxury of waiting till the end of the first trimester," says Marcy, the navy officer stationed in Georgia. "We're required to tell immediately." But people at work knew she wasn't dating anyone, and Marcy teaches young recruits. "My supervisor looked at me like, Were you sleeping with one of your students?" Marcy recalls. In general, most single mothers by choice find that upbeat and honest is the way to go and that secrecy backfires. At first Marcy didn't go into detail about how she'd gotten pregnant, as she was mindful of the conservatism of her colleagues. But don't ask, don't tell really didn't work for Marcy. In fact, it made the situation much more uncomfortable than it needed to be. "When a single woman says she's pregnant, everyone's wondering, was it a mistake?" Marcy says. Without an explanation, people don't know what to think. Even an unusual reality is less shocking and uncomfortable than letting imaginations run wild. And secrecy may only serve to alienate you further from potential advocates, as Marcy discovered. "One office mate was really uncomfortable," she says, "so finally I thought, You know what, I'm gonna go out on a limb here." Marcy explained the situation, and even showed him the donor profile. "I asked him, 'Does that freak you out?' He said, 'No, now everything makes sense.' He seemed relieved that there wasn't some sordid tale of a nasty relationship or unplanned pregnancy. After that, it was no big deal at all—he even turned out to be one of the few coworkers who visited me in the hospital."

All in all, Marcy concluded, "If you share the news with people in an upbeat way, it puts people at ease and makes it easier for them to be happy for you."

Coworkers are bound to be curious. "Everybody at work wanted to know who was the daddy," Alice says. "There were two guys at work who actually came out and said they were the baby's daddy." They were joking, and Alice just went with it. "I'd ask them where the check was," she says, adding, "It's not weird, so I don't let it be weird."

"We have a real gossipy, nosy accounting manager and she kept bugging the receptionist, 'Who's the father, who's the father?' " Cheri remembers. When Cheri finally told people the full story, one colleague said, "So, sperm donation. How'd that work for you?"

"She was just trying to show me she was OK with it," Cheri says.

Whether or not a single-mom pregnancy is any kind of a big deal at all can depend on the particular culture of your workplace. Ellen works in a progressive law office, and has lesbian colleagues who have already had kids. In fact, a lot of her colleagues have turned up pregnant. "When it was finally time for me to announce at work it was no big deal," she says, even though her coworkers knew she didn't have a husband or a boyfriend. "So do we know who he is?" one colleague asked, regarding the baby's father. "We don't? None of us? Oh!" It was a happy nonissue. And Ellen has not had a problem brushing up against the single-Black-mom stereotype. In fact, she has found the stereotype helps her feel less odd. "It isn't strange being a single Black mother. Some of the attorneys and the support staff are single Black mothers, and when all the lesbians at work are having babies, I wasn't the radical one!" Ironically, our nation's unfortunately high divorce rate helps single moms fit in, too. "Right now my family looks a little different," says Ellen, who has two young daughters. "But the divorces are going to start."

If you don't give people the full story of your pregnancy, or at least clue them in that you're thrilled to be having a baby, you may find that they fill in the information gap in a way you don't appreciate. Shortly after Samantha told her office she was pregnant, a Mormon colleague gave her a copy of her church newsletter, which featured a story on giving babies up for adoption. "Here's something I don't know if you've thought about it, but I thought I'd pass it along," the woman said. "I was really angry at first," Samantha recalls, though now she just thinks it's funny. "No matter how I became pregnant, at thirty-eight I think I could handle being a mom!"

## WHAT FRIENDS HAVE TO SAY

While most of the women I have spoken to had surprisingly positive reactions from their families, colleagues, and married friends, there are a significant number who have had hostile reactions from their single women friends. It's a topic that has come up in just about every Single Mothers by Choice meeting I have attended, and there have always been a few women who chime in and say, "That happened to me, too!" The women I've spoken to were uniformly surprised by it. The hostile girlfriends seem to feel as if, by pursuing a baby without a man, you're telling them they're chumps for continuing to wait for Prince Charming.

"One friend of mine is thirty-six and she's constantly telling me she couldn't do this," Cheri says. "But to others, she's saying, 'Should I be doing what Cheri's doing or should I keep dating?'"

One of Elisa's good friends dropped her when she got pregnant. "Her reaction was, Oh my God, this [having a child alone] is my only option, and she couldn't look at me and she couldn't be around me. We stopped communicating."

"I lost one friend who said she was really excited about it at first," says Samantha. The friend, who is single and Catholic, told her later that she had a hard time with it, and didn't think it was right. "My own psychoanalysis is that it's something she wouldn't feel comfortable doing herself, and she's envious," Samantha asserts.

It happened to Charlene, too. "That knight-in-shining-armor thing, it holds so many people back, it makes it harder to have friendships with other women. It just pushes us away from each other." Also, Charlene says, her getting pregnant as a single mom was an unpleasant reality check for some of her friends. "You're reminding me how old I am," they told her.

Another problem that several women mentioned to me is that, as a mom, they have been less available to their friends and their friends resent it, having gotten used to them being single and always available. "I was the caretaker, the mom," says Charlene. Now that she's mom to her daughter, she doesn't have the time to be mom to her adult friends.

"I was the Dear Abby of the third grade," says Jocelyn, who was thirty-nine when she became a single mom. She found that some friends didn't want their Dear Abby to have a daughter of her own. "I was emotionally supportive to a lot of people for a long time, and suddenly I wasn't as available, and they were upset."

You never know what kind of reaction you'll get. "One friend sent me a sympathy card after I'd had the baby," says Jocelyn, explaining that the woman assumed it was an accidental pregnancy and that Jocelyn was making the best of a bad situation. "I don't think most of my friends got it. The married ones didn't understand the single part, and the majority of my single friends didn't want to have kids ever."

But many women I spoke to had only positive reactions from their friends. "I've had support from everybody," says Melissa, the mom of twins, "though I do make a point of asking others what's going on in their lives, and not letting it be all about the babies."

Indeed, some single moms by choice find that they have become an inspiration for other women. "You become this conversation piece," Cheri says. One friend told her, "Oh, I was having dinner with this old high school friend and she's single and the clock was ticking and so I told her about you." When Jamie told her friends she was starting to try to get pregnant as a single mom, she says the more common reaction was, "Good for you, you're paving the way for me; I might be talking to you in a few years."

## INTERACTING WITH INSTITUTIONS: "WHERE'S YOUR HUSBAND?"

Before Scott was born, before the sperm I used to make him was even purchased, I thought about him—my future child—every time I filled out a medical or legal form. There it would be: "Father's Name." I'd fill in the name of my dead father who I never got to know. That's bad enough. But my child would have to leave the line blank. As an adult, there are not so many times you have to fill out forms like that. But as a child in school, there are countless instances.

What did not occur to me was what it might be like if, as a single mom of a child conceived through anonymous-donor insemination, you end up having to interact with big institutions and bureaucracies all the time. Like Amanda does. Her daughter was born a micropreemie, at twenty-six weeks and four days, so she was in the neonatal intensive care unit (NICU) for months. After about a month of staff members saying to her, "So, Mrs. Peters" (assuming she was married), Amanda, who has a sarcastic sense of humor, finally snapped. "When are you all going to accept that Mr. Peters is *not* stuck in the elevator and he's *not* going to be here shortly?!" She was able to bond with some of the NICU parents, but others were a problem. "This fundamentalist Christian couple were mortified when they found out I was a single parent with a sperm donor. The woman said, 'So, you expected this to happen?' As if I should expect this sort of thing since I did something so unnatural."

Meanwhile, even though she lives in New York City, Amanda still got the kind of reactions from hospital staff that you might expect in small-town Middle America. The hospital's birth registrar couldn't cope with the lack of a father. "There's nothing to put there? I'm going to have to see about this," she said. Then there was the staff's assumption that Amanda was a high-risk parent. "They sent a social worker to talk to me about single parenting: 'Do you understand the additional burden?' " Amanda, a successful forty-five-year-old professional, couldn't believe it. "Do you think I was in a trailer in Kentucky and just got pregnant with one of the boys in the back of the barn?"

Once Amanda's daughter was out of the hospital, the bureaucratic nightmares continued, because of the state agencies that provide the special services her daughter needs for her feeding problems and developmental delays. "The early intervention social workers are always asking, 'Where's the baby's father?' When I tell them, they don't know what to do with that. They have a whole second page of their form to fill out about the baby's relationship to the father." Some of them are good-humored about it, Amanda reports: " 'Got to ask you the stupid question,' they'll say." But many just don't get it. The worst, Amanda says, was the time a home-care nurse came to her home for an initial visit. The nurse asked Amanda, "Do you have an extra diaper for the baby?" Amanda said sure, and went to get one. "When I got back from the bedroom with a diaper, she had the baby in her lap with the diaper off and was literally inspecting her vagina," says Amanda, who was shocked and asked for an explanation. "I'm making sure you know how to clean the baby's labia," the nurse said, explaining that it was her job to make sure mothers know how to care for their babies—"especially single mothers," the nurse added. "Since you are a single mother, I have to make sure you're not so overwhelmed that you're unable to take proper care of the baby." Amanda was furious, and shot back, "Excuse me, Andrea Yates [the Texas woman who drowned her five children in a bathtub in 2001] had a husband—didn't work out too good for her, did it?" Then she asked the nurse to leave. "It's hard because as a single mom you don't have anyone to bitch to about the stupidity," Amanda says. "You enter this surreal government world, and every one of the federal and state employees asks, 'So, where's the father?' "

Amanda has sought out an online support group for parents of preemies, but that has its downside, too. Amanda noticed that a lot of the moms who were caring for their babies while their spouses were at work were writing things like, "If DH was here, DH would be fixing the whole thing." Who the hell is DH? she wondered. At last she figured it out: Dear Husband. And Amanda realized that for her, DH was not going to fix the whole thing. Perhaps he was stuck in the elevator.

## MAKE AN UNUSUAL CHOICE, GET A WEIRD REACTION

Like most of the women I've spoken to, I really haven't had any bad experiences telling people about my single-motherhood decision. But I've found that being open about choosing single motherhood can occasionally elicit some strange responses.

The most interesting comment I've gotten, for sure, was from a cab driver in St. Martin, where I was for an off-season, cut-rate Caribbean beach "baby-moon" (the last hurrah before the baby arrives—does it count if you go with your sister?) when I was six months pregnant. My sister had already gone to the airport to catch an earlier flight, so I was alone in the cab, and the young driver, noting my big belly, asked about my husband. I explained I was single, and answered his questions about how that all worked. "No boyfriend, either?" he asked, clearly shocked. "But you need a boyfriend to keep you open for the baby." I was uncharacteristically at a loss for words. He didn't seem to be offering his services in that regard, but he wasn't intending to be offensive, either. He was just genuinely worried about me and the difficult birth experience I would have. When I found my voice again I thanked him primly for his concern, but said that women whose husbands died or left them seem to get through OK, so I thought I'd be just fine.

Other than that guy, the only other truly weird reaction I got was from a pulmonologist I was consulting to see why I get bronchitis so often and how I could make it stop. Scott was about four months old, and I'd left him with a sitter. The doctor, a brusque New Yorker in his fifties, was looking at the new-patient form I'd just filled out and just could not seem to wrap his head around my single-mom status. The conversation went like this:

"You're single."

"Yes."

"But you just had a baby."

"Yes."

"But you're single."

"Yes."

"No husband, no partner?"

"Right."

"You're really single?"

"Yep."

"And you just had a baby."

"Yeah."

"Isn't that hard?"

I shrugged.

He paused and pondered.

"Are you gay?" he asked.

Startled, I paused as well. "Uh, yeah, actually."

"But you don't have a partner?"

"No."

"No partner."

"Nope."

"But isn't that hard?" he persisted.

"Actually, it's been a lot easier than I thought it would be," I said. After a few more go-rounds, we finally got back to the subject of my lungs.

# Can I Afford This?

I wasn't financially secure," says Frances, the personal trainer who has a young daughter as a single mom by choice. "I was scared to death. But I thought to myself, I can't afford *not* to do it. I wasn't going to let the fear stop me. And it's the best thing that I ever did in my life. Somehow the universe provides."

Anne, who is now the single mom of two girls, ages four and nine, felt the same way. "I wasn't sure I could handle it financially," she recalls. "But I knew if I didn't have a kid because of money, I would be so mad at myself for my whole life. It always works out."

For most women, choosing single motherhood is a big financial risk. But for those planning it in advance and determined to make it work, it usually does. "The universe will provide" is a common philosophy. But though money isn't everything, it is a very important consideration. Having enough money means that you will be able to afford things like safe and reliable child care, health insurance, and good medical care. Savings will help you and your child get through OK if you're laid off. And of course, money can often mean the difference between being a burned-out single mom whose life is always either work or child care, and a well-adjusted single mom who also has an adult life and can hire a babysitter from time to time. A great support system—grandparents who will babysit at the drop of a hat, for example—can make up for money, in some cases. It's ideal, however, to be able to rely on both a good support system and a decent paycheck. Most women I spoke to feel it's important to have some way of supporting the children they bear. But just how much money does it take, once basic needs are met? That often depends more on your attitude than on your bank account.

"If I worried about finances I would never have gone through with it," says Laura, who has twin sons and is currently out of work. "I mean, you've got to have a plan," she concedes. "But I don't think about it too deeply. Having a kid is not logical." But even applying logic to the situation told her to go ahead and take the risk. "People say, 'I can't afford it,'" she says. "Well, I can't afford it, either. But the fact is that people with a lot less money and resources than I have have more kids, and I don't see them dropping dead on the street, so there's got to be a way to do it. If I had less income, there are resources for cheaper child care. Now that I'm laid off, I've already signed them up for the city's free health insurance." Laura is not without resources—she owns her own building, so that provides some income. But even if she had fewer resources, she thinks she'd still have made the same decision. "I never considered it was a reasonable excuse for not having children," she says. "Really, how much money is 'enough'? I spent a lot of time growing up in a place where people are lucky if they have chicken once a week. I feel we live in such excess. Kids don't necessarily need Jumperoos and Exersaucers." In the end, she feels, the most important thing is love. "It would be worse to have gone through life without children than to have gone through it poor."

Jamie, who is trying to conceive, has a similar philosophy. "I'm not making a ton of money," she says. "But I'm not making twenty thousand a year, and I see women who only make that much and they make it work."

Most of the women I spoke to have pretty good incomes and so money is not a huge concern. Their financial independence was part of what gave them the confidence to pursue single motherhood. Still, knowing you have sole financial responsibility can keep you up nights. "I lie awake worrying about money," says Rachel, a single mom friend of mine whose daughter is a couple months younger than Scott. "I mean, we're OK, and there's nothing at all to worry about. If there were a problem, my parents are more than willing to step in and help out. But still, it's the hardest thing and my biggest concern."

Like Rachel, I've had my days of waking up in the wee hours with that stomachache of dread, worrying about money. I'm doing OK now, but what about the future?

Nina says finances were a huge worry for her in considering single motherhood. "I've had a long time to think about it," she said, since her doctor told her she'd better get pregnant before she was thirty because she'd need a hysterectomy. "At first I thought, no, I really don't want to be a single parent, I don't have enough money. But then I got promoted several times at work, and realized if I can't afford a nanny I'm not doing something right with my finances. I really *can* afford a nanny. Still, I held out as long as I could to save money."

## MAKING SACRIFICES

Worrying about money is often quite rational, even for those who are in good financial shape. A layoff, an illness in the family, and suddenly there are huge expenses and nothing to cover them with. Many of the moms I spoke to have had to make major lifestyle changes for largely financial reasons. Those changes include moving to a more affordable city, moving in with their parents, or just radically cutting their spending.

"At the time I became a single-by-choice mom, I had a high-paying job and I owned my own home. I didn't think I'd have any financial issues at all," says Mikki Morrissette. That all changed after September 11 and an unexpected job elimination while she was on maternity leave. Within three months, she had packed up her New York City home and moved back to Minneapolis. "It wasn't purely financial; it was a quality-of-life thing," Mikki says. She'd had the kind of job where she was working twelve-hour days when she was seven months pregnant. Changing her focus for the sake of her kid saved her sanity in a way. "Once I became a mom, my life just became much less stressful. My first year after my daughter was born, I just felt more rested than I had for years."

"I come from an upper-middle-class existence, the Buppie bourgeoisie," says Charlene, mom of five-year-old Tiffany. She, too, thought she was set financially, with a flexible job in nonprofit consulting. September 11 hit her hard as well. She ended up losing her job after a difficult pregnancy that turned out to be much more costly than she imagined. "Financially, I have been able to hold it together, but it hasn't been easy." She started her own company and has found ways to cut costs, for example, by enrolling her daughter in Head Start as a paying student, and by applying for scholarships to private schools, since she finds the gifted programs in the public schools to be even more white than the private schools are. It's been an education for Charlene, who wasn't raised in a way where she had to work the system.

Robin also thought she was set. But like several other women I spoke to, she unexpectedly lost her job while on maternity leave. "I thought it was no big deal," Robin says. "I thought in the few months I was gone, the contracting firm I worked with would just find me another computer-programming job." But when she was ready to go back to work, "tech was bust and there were no jobs." Robin spent more than a year looking for a new position and finally found a great one. But with her new concerns as a mom, she had to turn it down. "It was going to be ten hours a day and two weeks of training in Texas. If it was just me, a high-profile job like that would be great. But now I had this kiddo." Other jobs had other problems, like excessive commutes. So, after a year and a half of looking, Robin sold her house in Denver and moved back to her small Colorado hometown to live with her mom. At first the move was pretty crushing. "I was feeling defeated and depressed, like I was a teenager again." But Robin has been enjoying being a stay-at-home mom, volunteering for some nonprofits and retooling her tech skills toward teaching special education.

Indeed, part of choosing single motherhood is realizing that you may need to make major changes in your life. Jenny, an artist who makes money teaching and curating student art shows in corporate spaces, echoes many others: "Money is my biggest fear," she says. She has low monthly costs, since she bought her Brooklyn apartment years ago with the money her father left her when he died. Jenny hopes to stay put, but the apartment has appreciated in value quite a bit. "In my mind, it's my escape plan; I sell the apartment and move someplace else." Since Jenny doesn't have endless amounts of money, she realizes that she may need to change course. "I need a steady income; I can't live hand-to-mouth with a kid," she says. "If it means I have to go someplace else or find a full-time job, that's what I'll do."

"You realize you have the ability to make more money or to prioritize," says Eva, the New York social worker. She went to a few sessions of Debtors Anonymous as a way to get a low-cost financial-life overhaul before trying to conceive. "A friend wanted me to go to Costa Rica with her on vacation.

I didn't go, but I didn't feel deprived, because I knew that having a child would make me happier in the long run."

The need, or desire, to make different choices as a mom isn't just about requiring more money. Sometimes it's about wanting more time with your kids. Insufficient funds isn't Alice's problem—she makes far more than most of the women I spoke to. "I'm in a position where I have a really good salary," she says, "but it's a double-edged sword. Making a lot of money makes you want a lot of money. But right now I'm out of town on average one or two nights a week. It's not horrendous," she says, and it's mitigated by the fact that her son gets to stay in his own home with his grandmother. "But I don't want to waste my energy on work," Alice says. "I want to give my energy to him. I wish I had the courage to walk away from the money." Alice has thought about switching from corporate management to teaching. "But to go from a quarter million a year to fifty thousand a year is daunting."

## SINGLE MOM ON A SHOESTRING

Some single moms do manage to make it work on relatively low incomes. "I just put finances secondary and figured I could work out a way once I got there, and for the most part that's been true," reports Polly, a freelance graphic designer in Queens, New York, who has a seven-year-old daughter as a single mom by choice. Polly says she gets irritated when she hears women say, "You can't do this unless you make fifty-five thousand dollars a year." Yes, you can, she wants women to know. It will be harder, and you will need to be more resourceful, but it can be done, because she's doing it. It does require sacrifices, though. When she had her daughter, Polly moved back in with her mother, who lives in a state-subsidized middle-income housing project. Living with mom again is a mixed bag, says Polly, "but frankly, my attitude was, I want a baby and that's primary, so whatever I have to do to have this baby is what I'm going to do." She could have tried for a full-time corporate job, but she did not want that. "Despite being a feminist, I wanted to stay home with my baby." So at the beginning, she worked part-time from home, and since she was there to supervise, she hired a six-dollar-an-hour teenager to babysit instead of a twelve-dollar-per-hour nanny. She and a friend made baby food and shared it with each other so both babies had variety. There are a lot of inventive ways to save money, Polly says, throwing out a few: You can create a rotating playgroup, where five families get together and each family takes on the day care of all kids one day a week, leaving everyone with four days of free child care; you can share a nanny, or be a nanny; there's subsidized housing and even welfare and food stamps. "I've never had to do that, but I'm not opposed to it," Polly says.

Tauz, who's in her second trimester of pregnancy, also has a subsidized mortgage in which her payments are tied to how much money she makes. She has a background working in both banking and in foster-care administration, but right now she's back at school and is working part-time as a massage therapist. Still, she's preparing to welcome her baby to a cozy four-bedroom house on the Native American reservation where she lives, and she isn't too worried about finances. "Right now I make plenty enough money to support me and a child and still finish school," Tauz explains, though she worries about whether she'll be able to continue doing massage (her clients are in Santa Fe and Los Alamos, where people make "megabucks") into her third trimester. "I also have a really nice savings account, though," Tauz says, and once she gets her communications and psychology degree, she'll be even more marketable.

Angela, an old friend of mine, was a thirty-year-old cartoonist living in San Francisco when she decided to have a kid on her own. She really didn't have much money, just some freelance work as an animator and later doing lettering for mainstream comic books. "I decided to rely on the universe and the goddess and I'd just do what I could with it," she says. Angela ended up continuing to freelance from home, often working after her son was asleep, and saving money where she could. "Robin went to a co-op nursery that didn't cost very much, and I'd work there a few days a month," she recalls. "Some other people had older kids, so that's where his clothes came from, and we also got clothes at secondhand stores. A big freelance job came at just the time I needed to upgrade to a better stroller. It just all worked out." Angela was active in the local abortion-rights group, and she says it was her fellow activists who really pitched in to help her with raising her son. "They told me if you ever need a night off, we'll take care of Robin." It all worked out fine. By the time her son was in nursery school and her daughter, whom Angela also conceived as a single mom by choice, was in day care, Angela got into law school and got a fellowship to pay for it. She is now practicing law and has two well-adjusted kids, Jasmine and Robin, now fifteen and seventeen. Over the years, when I thought about single motherhood and worried about how it could work financially, I have always thought of Angela, who had so little and made it all work so beautifully. I still don't quite understand how she did it, but she sure inspired me and showed me it's possible.

"It's hard financially," says Shannon, the veterinary technician with the two-year-old, "because I've chosen a career that I think is noble but that doesn't pay very well. I had a lot of fears about the financial part, but I decided to hope everything would work out—and I haven't been evicted yet!"

Bonnie is a psychologist in private practice, so she is dependent on her own ability to work—there was no maternity leave or any of the other benefits of having a corporate job. "The year I had my daughter, I probably earned twenty thousand dollars. That was pretty horrible," she says. "I was sick some during pregnancy and I lost patients when I went on maternity leave. But I built my practice back up," she says, and she eventually started a side business. Bonnie's daughter, Grace, is now fifteen, and it has worked out fine, though she hasn't had the most expensive toys and clothes. "I didn't spend a lot of money on her when she was really little on stuff she didn't care about, because I figured the day would come when she would care, and that's been the case," Bonnie says. "We didn't eat out, we didn't go on vacation, we didn't buy fancy clothes." Now that her daughter's a teenager, "I buy her some new clothes," Bonnie says, but jeans and other basics still come from the thrift store. Grace has been OK with it, and so has Bonnie. "I like stuff," she says, "but stuff never made me happy. Grace makes me happy."

## IF YOU DON'T HAVE ENOUGH CASH . . .

Though many moms make it work, the risks of not having enough money are real ones. "Not being able to afford good child care is just devastating," says Elisa, who has a part-time job in sales. What she observed while shopping for child care was eye-opening. "I looked at one place where, while I was there, the caregiver hit a kid. But she was in a price range I could afford." Elisa would not leave her child there, but although the place she found for one-day-a-week care is "not harmful to your child," it's also not what Elisa considers ideal. But the thirty-five-dollar-per-day price tag is all she can afford. "The woman is safe, but she talks really loud and she watches TV all day. My daughter never watches TV with me, but now we argue about TV.

And she tells me what went on in the shows she watched; she just soaks it all in." Elisa doesn't approve, but feels that one day a week isn't going to kill her daughter. But she knows a married couple who sends their son to the same woman five days a week, and says, "I'd sooner live with her under a bridge than do that."

"Finances are more important than you even think they'll be," says Kimberley, mom of one toddler with another baby on the way. "As a single mom, finances are your only way to have that other person take care of something."

That's been true for Samantha, and it's affected her ability to have a social life. "There are a lot of single moms by choice who have nice incomes and can hire a babysitter whenever they want," she says. "That was never an option for me, and I don't have family nearby, so if I want to go somewhere it's an expensive proposition. Even just to do something after work, I'd have to hire a babysitter. I've heard of some people who have babysitting swaps, but living in the suburbs, it's hard to make that work."

There are a lot of single moms by choice out there who are living paycheck to paycheck, notes Debrah, who, as a surgeon, is not one of them. They make it work, she says, but it's a much harder row to hoe. "If you don't have money, you won't have the independence to do what you want to do," Debrah says. Her comfortable salary makes her single motherhood much easier. "I have the ability to visit my parents. We go on vacations. I don't have to worry about groceries, heating, lighting. And with my live-in nanny, I don't have to worry about who's going to take care of certain things."

## COSTS OF CONCEPTION

Never mind the cost of a kid—if you use anonymous-donor sperm and reproductive technology, just getting pregnant can cost a lot of money, and some wannabe single moms find that all the money they were saving for the baby is going toward making the baby. Part of Nicole's process of trying to conceive was saving money. "I cut a lot out," she says. "There weren't a lot of things to cut, but I did what I could," she says—downgrading from high-speed Internet and moving everything out of a storage facility she'd been paying a monthly charge for. "By the time I cut out all the twenties or forties or fifties, I had saved about two or three hundred dollars a month,"

Nicole says. "It's gotten a little ridiculous—I was shopping for a DVD player and I saw one at Wal-Mart for twenty-five dollars and I thought, I could do better. But I couldn't." In addition to working full-time as a publicist, Nicole took a part-time job to make extra money in the evenings. She had been setting some earnings aside, but that's all going to cover the twenty-five hundred dollars she pays monthly, out of pocket, for her medicated IUIs. "I know that financially I can only do this for so long before I run out of money."

The cost of trying to conceive "has been a big added stress," says Michele, who has been struggling with infertility. But her father has helped her out with some of the fifteen thousand dollars it has cost so far. "To him, it's investing in his own grandchild," she says.

When Lisa M. started trying to conceive, she had a good job, but then she became unemployed. "I couldn't put it on hold," she says. She had good insurance, though, so her COBRA covered most of the procedures. Still, it was expensive. "Out of pocket, it was probably between eight and ten thousand," she says. "And now I'm like, where would I ever get that kind of money? I work in computers, so I made a lot of money when I was young. I grew up a scrub on the streets of San Francisco. I didn't go to college. I never thought I could make the money I was making. At twenty-six I was making eighty-five thousand dollars. I never borrowed, I never had to take out a loan from friends or family." Lisa eventually got another job, but later got sick of the corporate scene and wanted to spend more time with her daughter, so she quit, went back to school, and became a massage therapist. She just recently went back to computer consulting. When she wanted a second child at age thirty-five, money was more of an issue and her insurance wasn't as good, so she decided to adopt through the foster-care system instead of doing the IVF she knew she needed to get pregnant again. Though the adoption was largely a financial decision, she's thrilled with her son, Kanye.

Once you have the child, though, it can put the expense of conception into perspective. "When I pop onto one of those online bulletin boards and I see someone complaining about the cost of buying sperm, I just laugh," says Rachel, mom of eight-year-old Frances. The cost of child care is so much more than that of sperm, she points out. "If you can't afford to get pregnant, you won't be able to afford the child." Rachel says she's found herself making "different life choices" than she would have thought. Previously, she owned a small bookstore and was happily living the hipster life in San Francisco. But, she says, with a daughter in tow, "I didn't want to rough it anymore." She ended up moving across the country, taking a higher-paying salaried job at Yale University, and buying a house. "You have to do this," she says—make choices that are different from the ones you would have as a nonparent—"or you're gonna sink."

## LEGAL "MUST-HAVES" FOR SINGLE MOMS

No one wants to sit down and plan for death. But making a will, naming guardians, and considering life insurance, while important for any parent, is crucial for a single mom. Who will take care of your child if you die, and how will they pay for it? There's no other parent to take up the slack when you get hit by a truck. My dad died of a heart attack at forty-two—a year younger than I am now. Much as I didn't want to consider it, I knew all too well I had to make sure Scott was well taken care of, both financially and emotionally. I made a will, chose guardians, and got enough life insurance to make sure it would not be a financial burden to raise him in my absence. Most single moms I spoke to were careful to do the same.

"My will was written before my son was born," Debrah says. "I have a living trust that's set up, funded by my life insurance policy. I have godparents for him—we had a long talk about how if I die, he goes to them. We discussed how Eric would be raised. I chose them because they're a very good example of how a couple interacts together, and they live in the same city as my parents so they would have access to him."

Creating a safety net for your child can be crucial, and setting up that net takes money or a willingness and ability to rely heavily on family, friends, and community—or all of the above. Like death and taxes, our dependence on the dollar is not something anyone wants to think about. The health, safety, and education of children shouldn't rely on how much money their parents have, but the reality is that they often do. So in considering single motherhood, it's fine to believe that the universe will provide, but your path sure will be an easier one if you're in a position to give the universe a nudge.

# The Daddy Question

I was on the phone to my mother one day and Scott, age five months, was "talking" in the form of the longest "aaaaaaaah" you ever heard, like an overzealous patient with a tongue depressor. He'd been "talking" for ten weeks, during which the aahs had just gotten longer and longer, indicating impressive lung capacity if not verbal skills.

"How about some consonants, sweetie," I said, and modeled, "ma ma ma ma ma. Mama!

"Yeah, right," I said in an aside to my mother, meaning, *as if*. She laughed and said, "They always start with da da."

I'm a reasonable person, so I was ready to compromise with "ba ba." For a week or so I'd been doing some carefully enunciated b-babbling, asking Scott, "What does the sheep say?" and singing, "Ba-ba-ba, ba-Barbar-Ann."

"Aaaaaaaaaaaaaaaaaaaaaah," he'd reply, or he'd just laugh.

The day after that talk with my mom, Scott finally put in a consonant. Guess which one. Da da da da da. I decided not to take it personally and da-da-da'd right back at him, and he laughed with delight.

In a 2006 essay entitled "Deleting Dad," syndicated columnist Kathleen Parker asserts that women choosing single motherhood are narcissists who think of children as accessories and believe that "men are only as good as their sperm count." I have yet to meet a single mom by choice who feels that way. Some do feel that one good parent can be even better than two. But most struggle, as I did, with the idea of creating a fatherless child.

"I was Daddy's Little Girl," says Ellen. "I had this really special relationship with my dad, and my daughters are never going to have that." Many women who choose single motherhood experience this as a loss—"I feel the father thing more than the partner thing," Ellen says—but they put it in perspective. "How many single moms are single *not* by choice?" says Jamie. "My kid will not have a father who left him."

"Will Eric have any long-term problems because he doesn't have a father? I hope not. I think this little kid will live his life and he'll have good experiences and bad, just like the rest of us," Debrah says. "What if he's one of those people who just has to seek out his biological father? I hope he doesn't, but if he does I would help him. I think I could find the identity of this donor, because I know where he lives."

"There's a lot of stuff in life that's not fair to kids," Nicole says. "I think it would be better for a child to have a father. But at the same time, there's a lot of bad fathers out there. Just because the father's in the picture doesn't mean it will be better for the child."

"Felix doesn't have a father, but I don't think that means he shouldn't be here. We have a great family life and he's a nice normal child. He can be sad, and I'll never know what that's like for him. But we all have something. Everybody has something that they're mad about at some point," says Kimberley, who was really impressed by a story Rosie O'Donnell told on TV about her son, Parker. "He came home one day and said, 'Mom, you don't know what it's like to have you as a mom!' And Rosie said to him, 'You're right, I have no idea. Tell me what it's like.' And I think that's the nicest thing you can say to somebody." If the child is loved and listened to, he's going to be OK.

"I think it's really important that he have a relationship with men. I want someone to give him that experience," Kimberley says. But at the same time, she thinks there are ways in which being a boy raised by a single mom can be great, citing the book *Raising Boys Without Men*, which looked at boys being raised without adult males around. It found that the boys were just as masculine as other boys, but also unusually compassionate compared to boys being raised in traditional families. "Men are so wrapped up in their child being something that they can relate to," says Kimberley. She feels like there's a possibility that, without that kind of pressure, her son might feel more free to be his own man.

Not having a dad doesn't mean not having a full family—or significant male role models, Charlene points out. In some cases, says Charlene, it can expand a child's circle of loved ones. "When my four-year-old daughter says her prayers at night, she doesn't just bless me and her grandparents. She has a whole long list of loving adults in her life."

"This doesn't mean that I've given up or that my baby won't have a father," says Jessica, who fully intends to get married someday soon. It also doesn't mean Jessica's baby lacks men in her life. "My stepfather has an incredibly special relationship with my daughter. More than anyone, he's totally enthralled with her."

Jenny, pregnant with her first child, agrees. "I don't necessarily believe that my kids are not going to have a father," she says. "I was able to get to a place where it felt OK for my child not to have one right now, or to possibly never have one." But that doesn't mean it's an idea she has given up on.

"I don't lack for male friends," says Laura, so she is not worried about finding male role models for her twin sons. She knows it's important, and she feels it's something she can easily provide.

Melle, whose three kids are by two known donors, has a perspective that's less focused on a single father figure. She feels that the nuclear family model is not good enough for any child. "An extended community plays a vital role in child rearing," she thinks. "Rather than my son looking up to one man, he has a variety of men to look up to."

Tauz, whose baby is due in another five months, wishes she could have provided her child with a father, but tries to put it in perspective. "I think of how many people I know who didn't know their fathers, and I know someone whose father is an addict and just caused a lot of pain. I don't think that not knowing your father would be the most devastating thing in your life, if you had your needs met and you were loved and you were safe and your mom was honest about it." She also puts it into a spiritual perspective: "My belief is that the soul of the baby chooses the parent. I think that it was my child's destiny to be born to a single mother, without a father."

Still, many of the women I spoke to were sad that they could not provide their kids with a father. Elisa, the single mom of two-year-old Skye, says she tries hard to be both mommy and daddy, but still feels there's something missing. "I look at Skye and think she deserves to be Daddy's Little Girl. She deserves to be loved in that different way."

Alice knows she can't be both mom and dad. "It's not like I'm a really girly girl," says the former U.S. army captain who served in the Gulf War. "But the guys take it to a different level, they take it where I've never gone. So I work to make sure that my son has significant exposure to men—though I don't always like what they do.

"My brother taught my son the elephant sound," Alice adds, as an example, and demonstrated a trumpet that sounded like a world-class nose blow. "And I'm like, *why?*" says Alice, suddenly gone from army captain to schoolmarm. "There are so many other animal sounds we could teach him, why the *elephant sound?*" Her brother also taught her two-year-old how to use the bathroom, again in a way of which Alice doesn't approve. "You know what he's doing? He's shaking his penis. He's two; I don't want him shaking his penis. He can sit down on the pot!" she said as I laughed, imagining droplets of urine going everywhere as her little dude concentrates on shaking it like the big boys.

There's still longing amidst the laughs. "When I see fathers with their sons, I covet that. I think that's a beautiful thing," Alice says. "Just like a mother with her child is a beautiful thing.

"Most of us want daddies for our children," Alice continues. "We want a lot of things for our children. And, heck, I want a husband. But I don't have one." Despite the missing elements, Alice says she is satisfied that her son is OK, and more than that, he has enough support and love to thrive and live a happy life. "Which isn't to say I don't have anxieties," she says. When her son proudly announced, "That's my mommy!" Alice says she was more nervous than pleased, "because the next step is, 'Where's my daddy?'"

Getting to a positive place was a journey for Alice, who started out feeling that choosing single motherhood was wrong. "I was against it for the popular reasons," she says. "Someone should have a mommy and a daddy. Having daddies in families is a good thing. You want the best for your children, and to me that's the best. And with that mommy or daddy comes a whole set of grandparents. It's twice as much support for the child." But Alice came to look more at the quality of the parenting than at the quantity of parents, and noted that there were married couples she felt shouldn't have had children. Meanwhile, she believed she'd make a great mom. "I felt comfortable that I had the ability, the resources, the emotional strength to raise a happy child."

I've always believed I'd be a great mom, too. But I know what it's like not to have a dad. It's damn hard. To this day, when I see a loving father spending time with his kids, I get teary. I never had that and I want it still. When I was in kindergarten, we sang "My Country 'Tis of Thee" every morning. "Land where my father died," I'd sing out. It made me feel sad, but also special, like the lyrics were written just for me.

"What does your father do?" kids at school would want to know. "He's dead," I'd say, as casually as I could, but still the kids would get uncomfortable. There were special father-daughter events from time to time. I'd either sit it out or bring a substitute. Most of all, there was that relationship I saw and heard about, the big protective daddy with the deep voice who loves you, gives you scratchy kisses, picks you up and swings you around, takes you out to the park, keeps you safe. I wanted that so much.

Sometimes I'd come up with this conspiracy theory, that my father actually *was* alive somewhere but that because of some scandal or some other complicated backstory, my mom had invented his death. Or maybe James Sloan wasn't my dad at all; maybe my mom had an affair with the milkman, and maybe *he's* still alive. The advantage of this made-for-TV-movie scenario was that it still gave me a remote chance of someday meeting my dad, and seeing for myself where half my genes come from. (Unfortunately, my resemblance to my dad's side of the family always pretty much torpedoed the milkman theory.)

I have no memories of my biological father, but I'm told we were close, that I was Daddy's Little Girl and that he adored children and children adored him, flocking to him like the Pied Piper. A family friend tells me that after he died I wandered around the house for weeks looking for him. "Where's Daddy?"

I'm sure my dad had his faults—sounds like he was a little on the wild side—but to this day when people who knew him learn I'm his daughter, their eyes light up and they go on and on about him. He seems to have been the kind of guy who inspired worship—an outsized personality, captain of the football team and an ace fighter pilot, a successful businessman who played as hard as he worked, was always the life of the party, telling funny stories when the evening got too dull. It was gratifying to hear all the stories, but painful, too, since he sounded like the world's most amazing dad, and I didn't get to keep him. And for me he will always be the perfect dad, since I never got to know him in all his human imperfections.

The closest I have to a memory of my dad came to me when I was thirty-five. It was a memory from when I was three or four, standing in the hallway of the tiny house we'd moved to after his death. I was wearing my favorite pajamas, the flannel ones with the tiny red-and-white checks. They had a white ruffled yoke embroidered with a red heart and the words "My Heart Belongs to Daddy." What I remembered through the heart of that toddler standing in the hallway was a feeling of loss—not the intellectual, conceptual loss of not having a dad, the one I felt quite often as a child, which was more along the lines of the pain of not having a ten-speed bike when everyone else does. Instead, this was the deep, intimate pain of having lost someone I knew and loved. In thinking about single motherhood, I was concerned that my child might have to experience that kind of sadness and longing.

My mom eventually remarried and had two more kids—my baby sisters—but no one stepped up to being the father figure for any of us. So my mother was, effectively, the single mom of four kids (with me as a helper), and she did a great job. She's loving and fun and strict and fair, self-sacrificing and giving to a fault. She's strong, independent, and capable. She taught us to swim, water-ski, drive cars and boats, paint houses, and hammer nails. She's certainly not perfect—who is?—but she raised four kids who adore her, who talk to her daily or weekly, and who visit her often. Most of all, despite all the ways in which I have disappointed and challenged her, I have never once had to wonder whether or not she loves me, and I have never once feared that she would abandon me. She really does love us all unconditionally. I have met so many people who cannot say the same about their parents. Based on my mom, I feel that a single mother can raise kids beautifully. I did not have a dad, but still, I feel lucky.

By contrast, I have been close to a number of people who had the perfect-seeming nuclear family and have spent the rest of their lives trying to recover from the damage. Like most people, I know of families that looked good on the outside, but that were physically or emotionally abusive and unsafe for the children involved. As much as most of us want to believe in the fairy-tale dad and in the importance of the father, child-abuse statistics prove that reality isn't always what we wish it to be, even if we haven't seen it for ourselves. I know of a single mom who married to provide a father for her children, and though she did get the approval of her family and society, behind closed doors she found she'd married an abusive monster. And I also have come to realize that it doesn't require blows to the head or verbal assaults to cause irreparable damage to a child. Perhaps the most damaged person I've ever encountered is someone whose mom and dad didn't like children but had four of them—because that's what they were supposed to do. In her picture-perfect family there was some parental behavior that could be construed as either excessive discipline or abuse, but the most damaging thing of all seemed to be a very simple one: lack of love.

## THE EXPERTS WEIGH IN ON DONOR INSEMINATION AND SINGLE MOTHERHOOD

Like me, all single-moms-to-be have different experiences and philosophies that inform and form their opinions. But how do the real kids of donor insemination turn out? Research consistently indicates that most kids of anonymous-donor insemination grow up happy and secure in families without a father present. Often their mothers' fears don't play out—having never had a dad, the kids don't feel the loss of one. Their alternative family structure is just a matter of fact to them. For me, this is wonderfully reassuring. Jane Mattes, a psychotherapist and the author of *Single Mothers by Choice*, says that to the extent that there's a problem, it's often traceable to the mom's attitude: "If the mother's comfortable, the kid's comfortable. If the mother's uncomfortable, the kid's uncomfortable. It's really, when you think about it, quite predictable."

Joanna Scheib is a psychology professor at University of California at Davis who studies the children of donor insemination and is the research director for the Sperm Bank of California. "All the research that's been done [indicates] the news is really good," she says. Scheib mentions a 2002 study that Charlotte Patterson of the University of Virginia did in conjunction with the Sperm Bank of California, looking at the adjustment of donor-insemination kids based on the sexual orientation and relationship status of the parents. Families headed by heterosexual couples, lesbian couples, heterosexual single women, and lesbian single women were all studied and compared. The study used standardized methods of assessing psychological adjustment, and also asked both parents and teachers to assess the children's adjustment. What they found was that there wasn't any difference between the groups in terms of how the kids were doing. What did affect the kids was

if there was any conflict in the family—for example, if there was dissatis-
faction regarding the division of labor between the parents. "The study found
that the structure of the family doesn't matter," explains Scheib. "What matters is what's going on in the family."

Scheib herself in 2005 conducted a study of kids ages twelve to seventeen
who have identity-release donors. These kids were all from Sperm Bank of
California donors, but the families are spread across the country. Overall, the
kids were positive and comfortable with their origins. Most shared their
donor-offspring status with those around them, reporting the reactions as
being neutral or positive. The majority were curious about the donor—
"What's he like?" was the number one question—but very few identified the
donor as an important person in their lives. "There are striking similarities
between donor insemination and adoption," Scheib says. "People want to
know where they come from." Interestingly, Scheib reports, "Adolescents
who were coming from households with single parents were the most curious about the donor's identity." She suggests that's because they have smaller
families, with no one on the other side, and that they don't have to worry
about protecting the other parent's feelings (whether the lesbian nonbio-
logical mom or the infertile dad) by pretending they aren't interested. Most
of the kids said they wanted to find out the donor's identity, but not necessarily meet him, and expressed a concern for his privacy. But in the six years
(since 2001) that the children of Sperm Bank of California identity-release
donors have come of age and had the option of seeking out their donor's
identities, only 25 percent have actually done so, Scheib reports. While the
kids of donor insemination seem to be doing very well, in general, Scheib
says "it's very important not to overlook the experiences of those who have
had a hard time." Some donor-conceived children, particularly the ones now
in their thirties and forties whose donor-conceived status was hidden from
them by their married parents, feel angry. "The first lesson is, don't keep
things a secret in your family," Scheib says.

Susan Golombok is the director of the Family and Child Psychology Research Centre at City University in London. Her 2004 study, "Children
Raised in Fatherless Families from Infancy," looked at the young adolescent
kids of lesbian and single heterosexual moms and compared them to the
kids of two-parent heterosexual families. The study found that lacking a father from infancy did not have any significant negative consequences for the
children. The only influence it seemed to have was that the children had

more severe disputes with their moms in adolescence, but the conflicts were within normal limits—the researchers suggested it may be because in heterosexual families the father traditionally tends to take on more of the discipline. Boys raised without a father showed more feminine characteristics, like being sensitive and caring, but no less masculine characteristics than the other boys, and their social and emotional development was normal. Single moms and lesbian moms did have a leg up in one respect—kids from two-parent heterosexual families saw their moms as being less available and dependable than those in fatherless families.

Peggy Drexler, a Cornell psychology professor who happens to be straight and married (and a mom) herself, studied boys conceived through anonymous-donor insemination who have single moms or lesbian parents. Drexler found the same thing that Golombok did: The boys were well adjusted, just as masculine as other boys but more communicative and empathetic. Her conclusion, as expressed in her 2005 book *Raising Boys Without Men*, is that "the number of times you eat dinner with your kids is a better guide to how well they'll turn out than the number or gender of the parents at the dinner table."

Nanette Gartrell is a psychiatrist based in San Francisco and the principal researcher of the National Longitudinal Lesbian Family Study. These eighty-four families and their children, who were conceived by donor insemination, have been studied since 1986. The latest follow-up was when the kids were ten years old. According to Gartrell, the offspring are well adjusted and not having a dad is not a big painful thing in their lives. Many are curious about their biological fathers, however. Interestingly, the kids who have the opportunity to meet their donors when they turn eighteen have more curiosity about it. "Two-thirds of the kids with permanently unknown donors are unconcerned about the lack of access, whereas one-third wish they had the opportunity to meet these men," Dr. Gartrell says. Perhaps, she guesses, this is because for the kids of permanently unknown donors, it's a done deal, and the lack of access is something that they've simply accepted. By contrast, half of the children who can theoretically meet their donors at age eighteen wish they'd already been able to meet him. But is this the searingly painful sense of loss that I fear it will be for my son, based on my own experience of losing my dad? Not at all, says Dr. Gartrell. "This is a mild regret, something that is mentioned occasionally, not a huge loss or absence."

Two of the single moms I spoke to have more than just a personal perspective on the daddy issue. For her book *Voices of Donor Conception*, Mikki Morrissette has interviewed scores of teenage kids with "choice moms," as she calls them, and donor fathers. The kids are definitely curious about their donors, Mikki says. But the overwhelming majority don't feel a painful lack of a father. Kids who have lost a father through divorce, death, or abandonment are traumatized, to be sure, and lacking a father for those reasons is terribly painful. But donor kids are coming from a very different place, Mikki has found. "If the relationship hasn't been there," she says, "it's really not that important to them that it would cause pain." That doesn't mean that there aren't mixed feelings, she says, and open discussion of the issue is an important part of making sure it doesn't become painful. "When the moms really are open about talking about it, letting the kids have their feelings, it doesn't become a problem over time."

Jenny also has a unique perspective on the daddy question. She was "very, very close" with her own father, who died when she was in her twenties, and so she wanted that kind of experience for her child. "I had to wrestle with the idea that my kid might never have a dad," Jenny says. At the same time, she'd also had a surrogate father since childhood. "My godfather was like another dad to me. That taught me that someone doesn't have to be your biological father to offer the love and nurturing and advice and all of that stuff." But what really opened her eyes was her experience working with the children of gay parents. Jenny's one of them—her dad came out of the closet and divorced her mom when she was a teenager. When Jenny was in her twenties, she was living in San Francisco and discovered that there was a whole community of kids with gay parents. She ended up working with one group, Family Pride Coalition, that organized a gay family vacation week in Provincetown, Massachusetts. Jenny was on staff for several years, leading workshops for kids ages nine to eighteen. Working with those kids, most of whom were the products of the "gayby boom," not children of divorce like she was, really changed her assumptions about family. "Some didn't have dads and some didn't have moms," she said, but that didn't seem to be a source of pain, since they were all extremely wanted children. "These kids, what they had and what they needed was just nurturing and love from their parents or parent," Jenny saw. "It didn't matter how many of them there were, it didn't matter their gender or sexual orientation, it just mattered whether or not there was love." Working with so many kids and seeing the same thing over and over again really helped Jenny later, when she started to consider having a kid without a husband or father. "Seeing how adjusted and cool they are, I realized that the intendedness of a kid outweighs whatever parent they might be lacking. All you hear from these kids is, 'Our families are normal, what's the big deal?' "

Jenny still wants a father for her kid (and a husband for herself), but she doesn't feel like not having one is going to be a terrible thing for her child. "I'm going to have to work harder to find male role models and uncles," she says. "I trust that my being conscious of the issue will alleviate any lack." And Jenny thinks that's actually a wonderful thing. Though she values fathers, she questions whether the nuclear family, with the wage-earning dad and the mom who doesn't work, is really the ideal situation for kids. "Because that model has become the standard, it's assumed that's what's needed, when more often it really isn't. There's a lot of isolation in that model. I think kids need more than just two adults in their life." As a single mom, Jenny feels she'll be motivated to help her kids create a wider community of mentors. "To me, if they are going to have three, four, five male role models in their lives, that's better than just one. It takes a village."

Lisa M., who has a ten-year-old daughter from donor insemination, experienced that kind of village. She grew up with the Filipino side of her family only, as her Puerto Rican father had taken off when she was quite young. Because she feels some connection to his ethnic identity, she chose a Latino donor, and she sought her dad out just to meet him when she was twenty, but other than that, he's really not a force in her life and she didn't feel like she was deprived. "My mom is one of seven," Lisa says. "There were uncles around, cousins around, we were a very tight-knit family, Sunday picnics in the park. I didn't have a dad, but I didn't miss him. Whether it's selfish or not, I have so much love for my daughter, that's all that matters. I have such a big family. I don't feel like she's missing anything."

Kristen, whose mother adopted her and her sister as a single mom by choice, says that she didn't miss having a dad. "It's hard to miss something you never had," she says. "I've had so many friends who went through painful divorces when they were kids and they really miss their dads. But I just don't have a sense of what it's like to have a father, because I never had one. What we did experience was so much unconditional love from our mom and our godmother and the whole family." Did growing up as the children of a single mom by choice harm them in any way? "I don't think so," Kristen answers. Both she and her sister are straight and have had good relationships, she says. "It hasn't affected our ability to relate to men." Kristen, who is tall, slim, and quite attractive, with light brown skin and long black curly hair, chalks up her wannabe single-mother status to bad timing in relationships and to moving to New York and getting absorbed in her career. Still, Kristen says, "I did weigh the decision heavily. When I walk down the street and see a father engaged with his kids, I think about the fact that I'm taking a purposeful action that will create a child who won't have a father." In the end, though, she thinks of her own experience and knows that what kids really need is "a parent who loves and supports them."

## HOW DO YOU TALK TO YOUR KIDS ABOUT THEIR FATHER?

Lisa M. remembers the first time the daddy question came up with her daughter, Mariah, who's now ten. "I was driving with her when she was about two and a half and she was in her little car seat and she said, out of the blue, 'My daddy is all gone.'

"I thought, I'm gonna have this conversation now? She's just a baby, where did that come from? What do I tell her? I pulled the car over.

" 'What did you say, Boo-Boo?'

" 'My Daddy is all gone.'

" 'Well, you get to meet him when you get big.'

She looked out the window and she thought about it.

" 'And when I get big, I can go to school?' And that was the end of it."

Lisa was proactive regarding the daddy issue after that, to get Mariah talking about it. "I would ask her, 'Do the kids ask you about your daddy?' " Her daughter would say yes. " 'And what do you say?' "

" 'I tell them he's not around, or I don't get to meet him until I'm eighteen.' "

One Father's Day, Lisa suggested that Mariah make a card for one of her uncles, but Mariah wanted to make one for Lisa. "That's fine," Lisa said. Another Father's Day, Lisa says, "she wanted to make a card for her cousin's bird; his name is Petie."

Debrah's son, Eric, is three, and is starting to talk about fathers. "He said, 'It's OK that I don't have a daddy, I have a Cathy and a Betty,' " Debrah reports. Cathy and Betty are a lesbian couple that Debrah has over for dinner often and he loves them, she says. "I think his interpretation of a daddy is 'people who play with me.' "

Charlene says, "I feel like I have to be honest with Tiffany about her beginnings, because I don't want her to be one of those kids who wakes up one day and finds everything was a secret. I tell my daughter she doesn't have a dad, she has a father. But that one day, if I get married, she'll have a daddy."

The most important thing, in talking about fathers with your kids, is just that—to talk about it, in an upfront and positive manner. As Jane Mattes, the psychotherapist, single mom, and author of *Single Mothers by Choice*, puts it, "If the child says 'lamp' and you say [in an encouraging voice] 'yes, lamp!' and the child says 'daddy' and you faint—that's not good. A child picks up on those cues from an early age." It's important to be comfortable with your choice, Mattes says, so you don't have to shy away from the topic of fatherhood.

There are books that go into detail about the best way to bring it up with your kid. *Choosing Single Motherhood* by Mikki Morrissette and *Single Mothers by Choice* both have great chapters on it, and the excellent book *Mommies, Daddies, Donors, Surrogates* by Diane Ehrensaft offers about one hundred pages on the topic. The consensus is to do it early, keep it positive, make sure you've dealt with your own negative feelings about having a non-traditional family structure, and make it safe for your kid to ask questions and have his or her own mixed feelings.

"I found a book called *Celebrating Families*," says Marcy. "I really want my son to grow up feeling like he's OK, and not feeling like a freak because of his family structure." For that reason, too, she has decided to start going on Single Mothers by Choice vacations, which are organized usually once a year, so her son will have friends who come from a similar background.

Though it's good to use technical words like "donor" or "father" instead of the more relationship-oriented word "daddy" for kids of donor insemination, you can't control what your child is going to come out with. "The first word out of my kid's mouth was 'Papa!' " says Robin, who used a known donor who is her on-again, off-again boyfriend as well. "I figure, what the hell, he's his daddy, I'm not going to sweat the details. He's figured it out. Kids are smart."

Laura has a double challenge, telling her twin boys not only about their sperm-donor father, but about their egg-donor biological mother. "I hope that ten years from now when they have to wrap their brains around it, it'll be a little easier for the general public to understand."

Liz's twin boys are three. "They do a lot of pretend," she says. "They've been pretend playing with a daddy and a baby, and I wonder if it's because they don't have to imagine a mommy because they have one." She explains to them that "some people have a daddy, some have two daddies, and some have one mommy."

Suzie, the Tennessee mom with two kids, has a unique perspective based on her kids' experiences. Her older daughter, Christina, has a dad—the abusive known donor who sued for partial custody—and her younger daughter Eliza has only an anonymous donor. Guess which one feels luckier? When Christina goes to visit her dad, she complains of the unfairness. And her younger daughter? "I thought she'd feel bad about not having a dad, but she doesn't want to have something as bad as what Christina has." And for now, Eliza seems to have "no curiosity at all about the donor," Suzie says, though she does enjoy hearing the story of how she was born.

Though the actual father of Suzie's daughter is a terrible father figure, she has found some good ones for her two girls. "My dad, my brother-in-law, and the nanny's husband are all father figures," says Suzie, who tells of skating and fishing trips that her girls have enjoyed with these men. Additionally, she makes sure her daughters are exposed to two-parent families that work. "I want them to see couples interact in a positive manner."

Kids in school ask questions, and Suzie tells of one example of how her youngest daughter has been able to take it all in stride. One kid told her, "You can't have children unless you're married, so you can't be here!"

"Eliza's like, Well, duh, I *am* here," says Suzie.

"Especially in the South, if you're a family that doesn't fit the mold of the traditional married couple, people don't quite know what to do with you," says Suzie. "They don't know what to tell their kids about our family."

I'd say that this is one of the many reasons to be open about your family structure. Provide people with the language they need, and model an upbeat attitude about it (more about this in Chapter 5). "The kids reflect the mother, at least until they're teenagers," says Jane Mattes, regarding the kids of the many single moms she has worked with. "Whatever the mother's feeling, the kid's feeling." If you have mixed emotions, it's worth working on the issue in a support group or in therapy.

Ellen, the D.C. public defender who has two kids, tells of the time the topic came up for her oldest daughter, Anna, two and a half, in day care. "Anna doesn't have a daddy!" another child taunted. "I intellectually knew it was coming," Ellen says, "but I was surprised at how hurt I was. I thought I would be more immune to it."

Though Ellen says it felt "heartbreaking" for her, little Anna was unfazed. "I tried to handle that particular incident casually but in a way that empowered Anna," Ellen says. "So when the little girl said, 'Anna doesn't have a daddy,' I said, 'That's right, she doesn't. What do you have, Anna?' And Anna said, 'I have a grandpa and I have Uncle Brad.' And I said, 'Some people have daddies and some people don't. Some people don't have Uncle Brads.' And of course the little girl says, 'I have an Uncle Brad!'—which is when I wanted to smack her. No, she does not have an Uncle Brad. But that's just how this kid is." Ellen says she thinks the incident didn't pack an emotional wallop for Anna, partly because the girl doing the taunting could just as easily have said, "I have a cupcake in my lunch and you don't"—it was just about having something that someone else didn't. But Ellen does talk to Anna about how lucky she is to have her grandparents and her uncle, and it seems to help her sort out the daddy question: "This past weekend, Anna said, 'I have grandparents and I have Uncle Brad, who does a lot of nice things for us. Daddies don't have hair. So Uncle Brad looks like a daddy because he doesn't have any hair. But he's not a daddy—he's Uncle Brad.' "

For Rachel, whose eight-year-old daughter already does know her sperm-bank donor and who seems OK with not having a daddy, being in contact with Frances's half siblings is a mitigating factor. "I always tell her how lucky she is to have two half sisters, so that whatever deficiency she might be feeling [about not having a dad] might be dispelled."

"My daughter is such a happy, well-adjusted child," says Diana, the professor from Des Moines. "It's very matter-of-fact for her. I've told her from the beginning about her story, and I joined Single Mothers by Choice specifically to see how other women dealt with the daddy question. On the group's Listserv, I was impressed by the idea that it's helpful to start talking to your child about her conception before she can understand it; that way the story feels like a natural part of her life, not something she had to sit down and be told about at an age when she was old enough to remember 'the talk,' " Diana says. "Also, if you start talking about it when your child is still a baby, you get to practice. You decrease your fear or anxiety and find that you have the language you need to help yourself and your child. It becomes a subject that you and your child can comfortably return to at different stages of development, as your child has new questions."

There are definitely some bumps in the road. "At about two and a half, my daughter thought my father was her father," Diana says. When she discovered that wasn't the case, "she was very upset about it." But that quickly passed, and she got it, Diana says.

"Last year, my five-year-old daughter and I went to a magic show at the Jewish Community Center," says Diana. The magician said he'd call on an audience member, and if they could answer his question correctly, they'd win a prize. Diana's daughter was chosen, and went up to the front of the auditorium. "To win the prize, the question was: 'What is your father's name?'" says Diana. "My daughter was onstage, in front of one hundred people, microphone in hand. My heart stopped." But to Diana's daughter, there was no crisis. "She just looks at him matter-of-factly and says, 'I don't have a dad.' To his credit, the magician said, 'Well, what do you know—I don't either. You win the prize!'

"I was so proud of both of us," Diana says. "On a stage, with a microphone—it's not going to get any worse than that. If she could tell her story confidently in that situation, I knew we were doing OK."

## SHOULD YOU JOIN THE DONOR SIBLING REGISTRY?

The Donor Sibling Registry has significantly changed the experience of having a child through donor insemination. Created in September 2000, it's a membership Web site that hooks up the parents and children of donor insemination (and egg donors, too) with the kids' half siblings, and in some cases with the donor himself. By early 2007, there were 7,685 paid members and 3,076 matches between siblings or children and donors. The Web site offers listings for sperm banks and fertility clinics all over the country, regardless of whether those facilities offer identity-release donors. (In fact, at present, the vast majority do not.) So now, part of deciding to become a single mom through anonymous-donor insemination is figuring out whether or not to join the Donor Sibling Registry. Most of the women I spoke to feel the way I do—they aren't quite sure what to think, but they'll probably join at some point. I also spoke to some moms who already have made contact.

"I'm in touch with the mothers of six of my daughter's siblings," says Amanda, whose daughter is only eight months old. They are all single moms, with the exception of one woman whose husband was infertile. "There's quite a variety of ages and lives and locations, but everybody seems pretty normal." And she sees a resemblance among all the siblings. Amanda is not certain what she will do with this information, preferring for now to wait to see what questions her daughter will ask, and what information she will want to seek out. And the anonymous donor? "A friend of mine is a private investigator and I gave him the donor profile, and he said, 'You realize within three days I could probably find him.' " Amanda is not interested. "If my daughter wants to know, she can embark on that." So why did she seek out the parents of her daughter's half siblings? "More curiosity than anything else," Amanda replies. She also thought it would be a good idea for the future, to ensure that none of the kids end up falling for each other. "I wanted to make sure we're not going to start our own nation," she jokes.

Charlene signed up, but feels a little wary. "If the donor contacts me, I will communicate with him," she says, but she will wait until her daughter is eleven or twelve to bring it up. She is not eager to contact the donor for a couple reasons—her donor is young and "I don't want another kid," Charlene says. Also, the ramifications of the biological tie are a little scary. "What if the donor dies in a tragedy, and he's the only child, and his family finds out he was a donor? How would I feel about them showing up on my doorstep, looking for their grandkid?"

Indeed, as much as I hated the anonymity going into this process, I feel that getting in touch with the donor could potentially open up a can of worms perhaps best left closed. In "DJ's Homeless Mommy," an essay he wrote for the *New York Times*, Dan Savage writes about his experience with open adoption. His child's mom lives on the streets, and has flitted in and out of their lives in disturbing and sometimes expensive ways. He and his partner ended up fishing her out of jail once. But even more disturbing are the times she goes missing. "As the weeks ticked by," Savage wrote about one of these times, "we admitted to each other that those closed adoptions we'd frowned upon were starting to look pretty good. Instead of being a mystery, [his child's mother] was a mass of very distressing specifics. And instead of dealing with his birth parent's specifics at, say, eighteen or twenty-one, like many adopted children, he would have to deal with them at four or five."

One hopes that the screening most sperm donors have been through make such distressing specifics unlikely. But the truth is that drug addiction, bankruptcy, mental illness, and bad health can happen to anyone. If your child gets to know the stranger who is his or her biological father, what happens if that stranger, now a significant acquaintance or friend, needs help? What will it mean to get involved? More important, perhaps, what message will it send if you don't?

Four-year-old Tiffany's questions were the reason Charlene ended up getting in touch with the moms of Tiffany's half siblings through the Donor Sibling Registry. Charlene and the other moms exchanged pictures of the children, and the moment that Charlene showed Tiffany a picture of one of her half sisters was an intense one. "It was a picture of a little white girl with blond hair and blue eyes," Charlene says. She and her daughter are African-American—Tiffany has toffee-colored skin and brown eyes—and the donor is biracial, Black, and Jewish. "Who is this a picture of, Tiffany?" Charlene asked.

"It's me!" Tiffany replied.

"No, that's not you, Tiffany," Charlene said.

"Well then, who is it?" said Tiffany, obviously struck by the kinship resemblance.

"It's your half sister," Charlene told her, amazed her daughter had seen herself in the photo.

"I was going to wait until Eric could decide on his own," Debrah says, but recently she'd become more open to the idea of contacting the other mothers and finding half siblings. "Maybe in the next couple years I'll contact them," she muses. "I'd like to provide him with some other relationship apart from me and his grandparents. That's part of the driving force to have another kid."

Suzie is in contact with the moms of some of her younger daughter's half siblings, but she has not introduced the idea to Eliza. "We were watching the movie *The Parent Trap* just after I was talking to one of the sibling's moms, and I asked, 'If you had a half sister out there, would you want to meet her?' And Eliza said, 'I have Christina, Mom, don't you think that's enough?'" Suzie is staying in touch with the half siblings' moms just in case, and she may bring it up in a few years. "The kids look a lot alike," she comments. But "it's given me comfort as a single mother how she reacts to things," Suzie says. "Kids think in ways that we don't anticipate."

Marcy was "delighted" to be able to locate her son's siblings through the Donor Sibling Registry. She registered and got an e-mail from a woman who has twin girls from the same donor. "Part of me thought, uh-oh, what if this lady is some weirdo," Marcy recalls. But then she saw the pictures of the girls, one of whom has the exact same smile as her son, who is now two and a half. "I think it's great!" she says. "It's a wonderful gift to be able to give him. I know there are a lot of things I can't tell him about his paternal heritage, but here's something I can tell him if he asks."

Meanwhile, Rachel and her eight-year-old daughter Frances have been in touch with Frances's half siblings all her life, since Rachel used Rainbow Flag Health Services, the sperm bank where the donors' identities are released three months after the baby is born.

"The sister relationship, to me, is a wondrous, beautiful thing. It gives Frances a sense of self. She loves her sisters. It's a mirror for her; she sees herself reflected. I was an only child, I didn't have that." One of the other mothers is a single mom as well. "She sends Frances a birthday present every year. It feels really natural to all of us. We made the conscious choice to use this kind of facility because we wanted the possibility of this community." The sisters visit each other from time to time and exchange pictures. In a way, it's probably a lot more positive than a more traditional sibling relationship, which would include fights and rivalry. But these half siblings with different mothers are just thrilled to have the sibling connection. "They long for each other," Rachel reports. "Whenever there's a separation, there's always tears." Rachel has heard stories of other women who buy up all of one donor's sperm so there won't be any siblings. Perhaps it's because of concern about possible incest later, she realizes, but Rachel finds it shortsighted. "A sibling," she says, "what a gift to be able to give your child."

# What About Sex?

*(Will I Ever Have It Again?)*

O K, I'm not going to lie to you. On a single mothers' Listserv I subscribed to when I was pregnant, there was a long e-mail back and forth about "buzzy friends." I don't think I've ever seen or heard such detailed discussion of vibrators—not even on the sex-toy Web sites that sell the darn things! These single moms got into where to buy them, where to hide them, how to deal with it if the kids find them, even recommendations regarding the best models to have on hand (the nonanatomical ones, naturally) if your kids are old enough to be snooping. Sure, many single moms and moms-to-be still manage to hook up with warm-blooded partners. But for most SMCs whose libidos remain intact, looking for love or sex becomes too logistically or emotionally complicated to deal with on a frequent basis. The solution? *Bzzzzzzzzz.*

That said, choosing single motherhood doesn't necessarily mean an end to your sex life. It just makes things more challenging—and maybe even a little more interesting.

## SEX WHILE TRYING TO CONCEIVE

There are still hard-core religious conservatives out there who would argue that sex should *only* be about trying to conceive. The rest of us admit that, most of the time, it's about love or pleasure—preferably both. Advances in birth control—and the realization that intercourse is not the only way to achieve orgasm—have helped us create and maintain the separation of sex from conception. Usually that's a good thing. But for single women who are trying to conceive with anonymous donor sperm, sex and conception can become separate to the point of absurdity—and confusion.

Take Michele. At age thirty-five, about a year after her decade-long marriage ended in divorce, Michele got pregnant by accident.

By accident? "Well, maybe it was a subconscious thing," she admits. "When I saw the positive home pregnancy test, I thought, That's it! This is what I want."

Michele decided to keep the baby, but not necessarily the boyfriend. "This was not by any means a serious relationship," she says. "I told him I didn't want involvement, and he was fine with that."

Unfortunately, that pregnancy ended in miscarriage. But it solidified Michele's desire to have a child before she got too old, and she figured "accidental" pregnancy was not the most responsible way to go. So she decided to become a single mom, looked into artificial insemination with an anonymous donor, and got started. On the weekend of her third intrauterine insemination she ended up on a date with the same guy who'd gotten her pregnant before. She hadn't seen him in a long time. "It was basically just a sexual relationship," she explains.

So, Saturday night, Michele used a condom with Mr. Booty Call. "He didn't stay over." First thing Sunday morning, she went to her doctor's office for an insemination.

"It was kind of funny," she says. And more than a little weird. Michele had decided that anonymous-donor insemination was the best way for her to go, and it was clear that her recreational relationship with Booty Call was not an appropriate foundation from which to create a child. Still, on a gut level, "it was kind of hard, because really my preference would be getting pregnant with him—being able to say, as the child grows up, 'That's where you got this characteristic from,' or if there's a health condition, being able to go to the guy and ask him if it's in his family."

Much like Michele, most women I've spoken to who were dating while trying to conceive kept their single-motherhood plans to themselves, unless the relationship became more serious. But even though keeping sex and conception separate under those circumstances makes perfect sense intellectually, sex is not an intellectual pursuit. And it can feel pretty bizarre, and emotionally confusing, to use a condom to protect yourself from the sperm of a flesh-and-blood man while paying through the nose to buy the same stuff from a stranger and have a doctor shoot it into your uterus.

Meanwhile, in another corner of SMC Bizarro World, for me as a lesbian sex and conception came a lot closer than I ever thought they would!

When I started trying to conceive in July 2004, I'd just separated from my three-year on-again, off-again girlfriend. Our relationship had been on the skids for a long while, but I loved her, she loved me, and I didn't want to face the reality that we'd tried and tried and it just wasn't going to work. In fact, as I lay for the prescribed fifteen minutes on the exam table after my first intrauterine insemination, I imagined her lying next to me, an infant nestled between us. It was a beautiful fantasy, and she would have made a great coparent—but the relationship wasn't quite right. The separation turned into a breakup about six weeks later.

By the end of September, I began seriously dating someone new—let's call her Jackie. I was completely open about my single-motherhood process, and she was supportive, but we didn't talk that much about it. It seemed way too heavy a topic to introduce into a new relationship. Four months and four failed inseminations later, I called the sperm bank and asked for my donor's pregnancy stats. They were terrible. Looked like he was pretty much shooting blanks. I started looking for a new donor, and in the meantime decided that I'd try to up my chances by adding a third insemination at home to the two I'd scheduled at the doctor's office.

When ovulation day rolled around, I was due to spend the night at Jackie's apartment. Some people will freak out if you bring your toothbrush over to their house too early in a relationship. Meanwhile, Date from Hell, I asked her if it was OK for me to bring my nitrogen tank full of semen— and, by the way, would she be willing to help with the insemination? After so many sterile medical procedures, I was aching to have this conception attempt be a shared human experience. Jackie was nervous about it—we'd already had our ups and downs, and she was worried she'd feel responsible if I didn't get pregnant, or worse, feel responsible if I did—but I reassured her that I just wanted company, and she ended up agreeing.

As always, it was a messy procedure, with some of the semen spewing out of the airplane-pressurized vial onto my fingertips as I unscrewed the cap. I drew the remainder into the syringe (Jackie snapped a souvenir photo), handed it to her, and lay back against her pillows. After the deed was done— it takes all of two seconds—we lay together on the bed and things started heating up. One thing led to another, and we ended up having some pretty spectacular sex.

It felt perfect. I was more in love than I'd ever been in my life, and despite some challenges I was really hopeful about our relationship. The sex was amazing, everything about her was amazing, and here I'd just had a shot at conception the way I'd always wanted it—at home, in love, in bed, through sex. Then I remembered what had just been on my fingertips. Oh, shit.

I was scared and horrified as I told Jackie what we'd just risked: the first-ever bona fide accidental pregnancy from lesbian sex. Absurd—but eminently possible, given the circumstances. I apologized profusely and pledged full child support. She took it pretty well, considering how hugely irresponsible I'd been. Meanwhile, I was secretly delighted and hopeful. I'd been kidding myself when I'd told her the insemination was not going to be a Significant Relationship Moment. I was so in love, and I imagined how beautiful Jackie would be, pregnant with what could only be construed as our child. Her slim body became ripe and rounded in the soft-focus video in my mind. There was probably a sunset and a field of flowers in there as well. (No, being gay does not exempt you from romance-novel fantasies, though it does perhaps highlight their ridiculousness!)

That was Saturday night. Like Michele, I got up early Sunday morning to go to the doctor's to be inseminated again—first kissing my possibly pregnant girlfriend good-bye and leaving her to sleep in.

Alas, Mr. Shooting Blanks didn't do it for either of us. After one more cycle, I dumped that donor. Shortly after that, Jackie dumped me.

When Nicole first started trying to conceive, she pulled her online profile off the dating Web site. "I initially felt that I could not be dating and trying to get pregnant at the same time," she explains. "I did not think, ethically or morally, that I could be dating one person and trying to get pregnant with another. And I didn't think I could commit myself wholly to getting pregnant if I was still dating." Once she started the process, she was surprised to find her opinion evolving. "I realized I don't need to meet someone to be a mother; I'll be a mother either way." And friends encouraged her to date. So, Nicole says, "I reposted my profile online." This was all very recent, when I spoke to Nicole, and she still was not sure how well it was going to work. "I feel I need to be honest about it from the beginning, but I'm afraid it will scare off 99.9 percent of the guys out there. A lot of people are still shocked by the idea of becoming a single mom. They definitely come around real quick, but in a dating situation, I'm not so sure.

"Then there's the practical side of it. How would you know it was the donor's baby and not your date's? That would be the biggest worry: Who's the author?" Nicole laughs. "It would seem so strange to put on a condom while trying so hard to get pregnant."

All that aside, Nicole says, "It's kind of fun to be back in the game again, because ultimately I would love to meet someone, fall in love, get married, and have kids."

## "HONEY, I'M PREGNANT!" (AND IT'S NOT YOURS . . .)

Men can get a little weirded out when they find out the woman they are dating is trying to get pregnant with another man's sperm. When they find out she *is* pregnant, it can get even weirder.

Cheri met a new guy right after her third failed intrauterine insemination as an aspiring single mom. She took a monthlong break from trying to conceive, mostly to take stock of the failure, but "I considered tabling the whole thing, since the relationship had possibilities." Instead, after her break, she started up again—and wound up pregnant.

"It was awful!" recalls Cheri. "My boyfriend and I had been dating three months, and I had not told him about my SMC pursuits. We were having sex, which made it more complicated because when I told him I was pregnant, he thought, Oh my gosh, I am the father of this child." He wasn't. "To make things worse," Cheri says, "I told him over the phone!

"I remember a friend being pretty rough on me at the time, when I told her I hadn't told the man I was dating that I was trying to conceive. She said,

'You're playing with fire.' But in my head, I felt OK not telling him earlier," Cheri says. "The insemination process really zapped a lot out of me. My body really craved that physical comfort [of sex]. If anything, I was using him for the comfort and closeness, not to get pregnant." But in retrospect, Cheri wishes she'd been more honest. "I was justifying that I wasn't lying, but I wasn't being truthful, either," she admits. "I regret that."

Cheri's boyfriend took it pretty well at first. "The next time we saw each other and he was kissing me good-bye, he said, 'I've never kissed a mama before.'"

But then Cheri's hormonally charged first trimester took its toll on the relationship. "I was insane," she says. "I was crying all the time. Everything seemed traumatic and big. It was a cold winter, and even the cold would make me cry. It was a roller coaster—and a couple of times I took it out on him."

The abrupt swings into sadness lasted three months, and then "I hit the second trimester and I felt like Mary Freaking Poppins—I just wanted to dance and sing, I was so happy," Cheri remembers. But it had all been a bit too much for her boyfriend, who hit the road at about the same time that the show tunes commenced.

For some men, however, a woman's choice to have a child on her own works out just great. How often does a guy get to have a purely recreational sexual relationship with a woman in her thirties who wants to have a kid?

That's what happened to Melissa. At thirty-four, she left her marriage to a man she'd been with for ten years because of the childbearing issue. "I thought we'd agreed to have children," she explains. "I was willing to compromise on a lot of things but not that." By thirty-eight, she'd started on Plan B—in vitro fertilization with anonymous donor sperm. All systems were go, but then Melissa got a job offer and started dating a new guy who lived a couple of hours away—and it was going well. She thought about putting Plan B on hold for a few months, but then saw a news report on embryo freezing. "I decided to go through half an IVF cycle and freeze the embryos," she says. That way, she figured, she'd take the pressure off the relationship and buy some time to settle into the new job. Then, at the last minute, she decided to implant a few of the embryos after all, and she ended up pregnant—with twins.

"When he heard I was pregnant, he thought it was by him," Melissa says. "I was so surprised when he stuck around!" But he did, and the two of them were "having fun" up until about two weeks before she gave birth. There wasn't even much talk about her pregnancy: "It was the elephant in the room. It didn't come up." Turns out he wasn't really interested in marriage, "but sex, definitely." And that suited Melissa just fine. "This guy, I like him a lot, but he isn't my focus. And that's made for a better relationship." Before she got pregnant, Melissa says, "I'd be thinking, how can I get this man to fall in love with me and marry me and have children with me? That was all I cared about." Now Melissa says she'd love to get married again someday, but "it's not all-important anymore."

And the sex? During pregnancy it was great—just what she needed. But when I talked to Melissa, the twins were eleven weeks old, and though sex was still on her boyfriend's mind, it wasn't on hers anymore. "Mostly he just wants phone sex and I just can't deal," she says. "I'm living temporarily with my mother, there are two screaming babies in the next room, and I haven't slept. To his credit, he's calling me—I just don't have time to call him back."

## SEX & THE SINGLE PREGNANCY

Melissa was one of the lucky ones. While some women keep dating, especially in the first trimester, dating after that test stick turns can get awkward. "You have to do all this disclosure right off the bat, which was weird," says Anne, who went on a few dates at the beginning of her pregnancy. "I was having dinner with one guy in an Italian restaurant, and he nearly spit out his wine he was so shocked!" Most pregnant single moms by choice end up staying home alone (with their buzzy friends).

It can be awkward, even if your date isn't shocked, because you've basically got a runaway freight train in the form of the fetus bearing down on the relationship. Liz, another lesbian single mom, got involved with someone right after she got pregnant, and they stayed together for two years. "It was a bad idea," Liz says. "I tell friends who are considering having a baby on their own to stop dating. Everything becomes confused. How do you date someone without getting them involved in the process? There's an urgency; you're wanting to figure everything out before the baby comes." Liz and her girlfriend ended up moving in together, but split when the twins were close to two years old, partly because, Liz says, her girlfriend "wasn't one hundred percent into having kids."

Pregnancy causes a big drop in sex drive for some women, and there are many who just feel too fat, awkward, nauseated, or uncomfortable to want sex. For these women, being single can be a godsend—no spouse to invent headaches for or feel guilty about. And for some, the idea of going out on a date with a bun in the oven just sounds crazy: "Oh, God, no!" said Jessica, a self-described *Sex and the City*–style single mom suddenly gone proper. "I think it would be really weird for someone to date a pregnant lady." But for many others, sex drive increases dramatically, due to the surge of hormones, and being single can be pretty frustrating.

"It was horrible!" remembers Marcy, now the mother of a two-year-old. "When I was pregnant, all I could think about was sex." This, after a lifetime of low sex drive. "It just seemed like such a waste," she says, adding, perhaps only half-jokingly: "If I had felt this way earlier, maybe I would have gotten a husband!"

On the upside, orgasms in pregnancy can often be more intense—and that's true no matter who gives 'em to you. "Let's just say I went through a lot of batteries in those nine months," one single mom wrote to the online community.

One pregnant single mother by choice actually came up with a medical excuse for buying—and playing with—sex toys in her third trimester. There's a midwifery technique called perineal massage that, if done consistently in the last month of pregnancy, is supposed to help make delivery easier, lowering the risk of tearing the perineum (the tissue between the vagina and the anus) and avoiding the need for an episiotomy.

"You're supposed to put your thumbs in your vagina and press down toward your anus, stretching the tissue until it burns," Ginny explains. "First of all, that's hard to do to yourself, especially when you have a giant belly to reach around. And secondly, what fun is it?"

Instead, figuring she could add some pleasure to the pain, Ginny paid a visit to her local sex-toy emporium and bought herself a few different sizes of dildos—including the absolute biggest, thickest one they carried—and a big bottle of lube. Night after night, she eased her way up in girth. "It was uncomfortable, sometimes painful at first," she confides, "but using a vibrator at the same time helped, and once I got it in, it felt amazing!" She was able to stretch her perineum and have one of those intense pregnancy orgasms as a reward every time. (One plus to being single: a standard-size male partner might have felt more than a little threatened by Ginny's outsize silicone playmates.)

Sex aside, pregnancy is a profoundly physical experience, and it can be hard to go through it in a vacuum of touch. In addition to a possible increased sex drive, pregnancy brings on physical changes that many single women would love to share with an intimate partner. For example, like many women, the minute I was pregnant my breasts became unrecognizably large. In the course of a month, I went from a barely-B to a full-on D-cup. While I wasn't so thrilled about the hard-core support I now needed (my well-endowed friend Sally had to teach me the "wear two bras at once" trick), I knew the change would likely appeal to a partner. It was sad not to have someone to appreciate the changes the Titty Fairy had wrought. (Though once, I had a guy literally hold an entire conversation with me while staring at my new cleavage. Since this had never come even close to happening to me my entire life, I found it more amusing than insulting.)

It's not just breasts—as my belly expanded and the baby started to kick, there was also no one to marvel and enjoy it with me. Most people either didn't feel comfortable touching my belly, or they just weren't all that interested in whether or not the baby was kicking. (Scott's first kick happened late one night when I was going home in a cab after dancing. I let out an involuntary "Oh!" of surprise and then had to explain myself to the cab driver, who was like, "Whatever, lady.") There was one guy I'd swing-dance with who would occasionally lead a move by placing his hands on my hips or belly—a perfectly acceptable but somewhat uncommon type of dance lead. Every time he did it, I was thrilled. Something about having someone else touch my changing belly made the pregnancy experience more real, more complete. It wasn't sexual at all, but it was a sensual relief to finally be touched there. For a long, long time, he was the only person who ever did. He was someone I barely knew, but in an odd way he turned out to be an important relationship for me as a single mother by choice.

Later in my pregnancy, I was lucky to have an old friend take an interest in the baby. Each time she came over she'd insist on trying to feel him kick, and, unlike most others, would wait patiently with her hand on my belly until he actually did. She was the only person in my life who did this, and it meant so much to me to be able to share the baby's movements with someone.

For me, these little things were significant and helped me through the sadness of being alone. But there were other sensual needs that just plain went unmet. In my third trimester, as my shirts got hiked up higher and my pants got belted even lower, I'd sometimes find myself absently touching the exposed soft curve of skin under my firm pregnant belly, right above the bikini line. It was a really sexy little spot, like the nape of the neck or the small of the back—but I was the only one to discover it.

Personally, my sex drive didn't decrease due to pregnancy (I wish it had!), but it didn't get stronger, either—thank God. And I was fortunate to have a number of women interested in dating me, despite (or perhaps because of) my pregnancy. I suspect that gay single moms may have it easier in this regard. I don't know if lesbians find the pregnant body sexier than straight men do, but at the very least they don't have paternity and child-support fears to contend with. Plus, being women, some may actually be attracted by the possibility of an insta-family.

Unfortunately, despite an aggravatingly intact sex drive, I did not respond to any of the opportunities I was presented with—I was still in love with my ex, Jackie, who'd dumped me five months before I got pregnant. The result of my idiotic pining was a lonely and nearly sex-free pregnancy. The only time I had sex was at about six weeks, with Jackie, during what was for her an isolated afternoon of backsliding. It was both wonderful and heartbreaking for me, since I wanted her back as my girlfriend, not just for a roll in the hay. I can't speak for how she processed it emotionally, but I can tell you that she did indeed enjoy my new "implants." Hey, at least they got a few minutes of saucy X-rated action in the nine months before they became a G-rated food source.

Robin had a sex-free early pregnancy, but that changed as she got closer to her due date. After conception, she kept seeing her off and on *"que será, será"* boyfriend, who was, as it later turned out, the father of her baby. But for the first six months, "he was off working in California and I'd just hear from him occasionally," Robin says. "I didn't have anyone to cuddle with." Then he came back. "I kind of liked having him around," she says. "It's kind of an unnatural state to be pregnant and alone. It was nice to have someone appreciating my body—he liked the fatness. And just having someone to say to: 'Put your hand on my belly and feel that—pow!' Sex during pregnancy was pretty nice—a lot of that stuff was a lot more sensitive, and it was more intense. I think it's nice to have an appreciative fellow around at that time."

## WILL SINGLE MOTHERHOOD PUT A STOP TO SEX—AND LOVE?

Even if they didn't lose their libido during pregnancy, many women lose it in the aftermath of birth, or simply lose interest because they are so in love with their babies. For a single mom, this can be good news. Bad news is, this might not turn out to be you.

"Since I had my son [now age two], I don't really think about sex anymore," says Marcy. "I don't feel like there's anything missing in my life. Relationships are a lot of work, even if it's with a good guy. Then if he has issues, it's even more work!

"I'm not a man-hater by any standard," Marcy continues, "but I really feel completely fulfilled by having a child. I kind of feel like I cheated, in a good way, because I got to have the baby without having to find the man first. I feel like the cat who swallowed the canary."

Suzie, who has two daughters, ages eight and ten, doesn't date, either, and doesn't miss it. "If you're in a relationship you have to devote a lot of time and energy to it. I don't want to take the time away from my kids." Realistically, it would be hard to fit in. "I manage a large number of people at work, and all the kids' school activities, and the two dogs and the pet rat and the house," she says.

Jocelyn says she hasn't really dated since her fifteen-year-old daughter was born. "I had put so much energy into relationships and worked so hard, with so little gain. I didn't see how I could focus on a relationship, since they are so time-consuming, and focus on this child, so I didn't seek out a relationship." For her, it was a welcome shift. "I'd been single and dating or married and miserable for twenty years. I felt that was enough time. It had been fun, but I was glad *not* to focus on myself and my life."

On the opposite end of the sex-drive spectrum, "I was climbing the walls in the hospital, four days after giving birth!" one supercharged single mom admitted to the Listserv. She was tempted to take matters into her own hands, she says, but was afraid someone would "know," or worse, that she'd be caught. So she waited until she got home to become "master of her own domain," as she delicately put it.

Most women probably find themselves somewhere in the middle ground between celibate and sex-obsessed. But, according to many single moms (married ones, too, for that matter), the loving, cuddling, constant physical attention they get from and give to their kids really does take the edge off.

"It's hard to describe the intensity of the tactile pleasure you get from a baby or a child," says Anne, whose daughters are now four and nine. "I just love touching my children. It's not sexual at all, but it's something you don't experience with your friends. It's a type of touch you otherwise only experience with an intimate partner. It's really taught me how deprived we are in our touch-phobic society!"

It's a lovely, cozy, animal feel, indeed. Snuggling with baby Scott satisfies some of that longing I've always felt peering into the hamster cages at the pet store, seeing the whole hamster family snoring cozily, piled on top of each other in the cedar shavings. I miss having a mate, and having sex, but I have this soft, warm, snorting little creature who, when I am curled around him, kneads my belly with his feet, like a kitten, and nurses greedily. Sometimes he'll even reach up and softly stroke my cheek. It's hard to get desperately lonely with a companion like that.

Baby love only takes most gals so far, though. "I rarely sit around and think, Oh, I wish someone were here to help me make bottles or do laundry," one single mom of an infant reports. "But I do sit around often and think, I wish I could fall asleep in someone's arms tonight, or I wish I had someone to make out with."

Finding someone to make out with after having a kid can take some doing. Suddenly, you can't be as spontaneous—an evening out takes careful planning and scheduling, and might have to be scrapped at the last minute due to your kid's ear infection or stomach flu. "It's closed the door on that carefree kind of 'Oh, I'm gonna throw on that hot little outfit and go out to a jazz club tonight' sort of thing," says Cheri, mother of a two-year-old boy. "Everything about leaving the house is totally planned." And, once their children are past infancy, most single moms are very careful about who gets to form a relationship with them. "My parents were divorced," says Liz, the single mom of three-year-old twins, "and I can remember the random guys wandering in and out." She is determined not to make that same mistake. "I'm not going to invite someone in to coparent after five minutes," she adds. And as a working mom, her kids are her priority in off-hours. As a result, in the love-life arena, "there are tremendous time constraints."

There's also a dating downside to being an older mom that several of the women I spoke to mentioned. "Men who are my age, their kids are out, or going out the door," says Charlene, who is forty-six. They aren't interested in dealing with young kids again. "You go out on a date with someone and he's fine, and then you talk on the phone later. When they hear that four-year-old in the background you don't hear from them again." But for a woman in her mid- to late forties, she says, "dating someone younger, that doesn't work because they *want* to have another child." In addition to the age issues, Charlene also is concerned about protecting her daughter and protecting her family time. "You meet for lunch," she says of her dating strategy. "And men get attached too quickly and they want to be in your life. I'm like, I've got to get to *know* you."

"Once you have kids, you're a lot more careful," says Anne. "If you were a person who liked to have one-night stands, that's over," she says—"unless you're so together you get a babysitter, go to a bar, and know where to go . . . but that's taking chances with your own personal safety, and you just don't do that when you're a mom." And it can be a challenge to find a date. "Guys my age want to be dating women in their twenties," says Anne, who is forty-two. Also, for some guys, single mothers by choice are not exactly a turn-on, Anne says. "Women who choose to do it themselves are really powerful, strong women, and that can be intimidating to men. It's almost like we're untouchable." Then, she says, single moms have to be even more assertive in the dating arena because of logistical issues—they don't have time to waste; the babysitter clock is ticking. And though many men claim to want an aggressive, assertive woman, the reality is that many don't want their date to take control.

Then again, once you have a kid, you may find that you're a lot pickier. "Sex was such a big part of my life before," says Kimberley. "And I'm totally open to dating. I like myself, and I like myself more as a mom. People ask me, 'Oh, won't it be baggage?' But I don't think of kids as baggage." Still, there's a difference for her in thinking about dating. "Now that I have a child, there's this added piece of, Who is good enough for me to put into my son's life?"

Debrah, who has a three-year-old son, discovered the hard way how complicated it can be to combine a relationship and single motherhood—if it's the wrong relationship, it can be a bad scene. At first, she had thought the two wouldn't mix. "If I was going to have a child and raise him on my own,

I guess I figured that if there were going to be any romantic relationships, it would be after the child was grown." But since her son was born, Debrah dated one guy for a couple months, and then ended up in a ten-month relationship with a guy who was her night nanny. That was a disaster. The relationship became very "full of turmoil," she says, and it was difficult to extract herself from. "I had started to allow this guy to call Eric his son, and I still get cards from his family saying I'm a bad parent because I won't let them see their 'grandchild.' I think I was very vulnerable, and he and his family had me convinced that any father was better than no father at all." In order to get out of the relationship, she had to line up another nanny. She ended up asking her parents, who lived far away, to come out for two months so she could sort it all out. Since then, she's been concentrating on her successful surgical career and on raising her son. "I'm not in any social circles where there are single men," she says. She doesn't feel her life is lacking much anyway. "My life is very full right now. I like what I do, and I like my time with my son. Having a child is a lot more entertaining, more fun, more full of joy than I thought it would be," Debrah says.

Single moms also get pickier about how to spend their precious downtime. "If I have time for me," says Laura, who has two kids, "I don't want to spend it on someone who might be boring, or worse." It's a financial consideration, too: Is this date going to be worth the thirty to fifty dollars you'll have to pay the babysitter, in addition to any transportation, meal, and entertainment costs? "If you're going out with me and you cancel at the last minute, you ain't never going out with me again," cautions Michele, " 'cause that costs money!"

Many single moms by choice go the online dating route, since meeting people that way can be done at home, after the children are asleep, and you can screen out the really bad matches before even leaving the house—or so it goes in theory. Others get by, maintaining "friends with benefits." Anne, the single mom of two, says, "I think it's really easy to just slip out of it. It's a choice of mine not to be as sexually active as I could be. For me it's easier to just sleep with old friends once in a while, or to get more out of masturbation."

It also really makes a difference where you live, unfortunately. Anne moved from San Francisco to a small town in California. "I had this kind of small-town reality check," she says. She went out on a date with a divorced guy who had two grown kids and had been married thirty years. "He could not understand the whole sperm donor–single mom thing," she says. "I just thought, Oh, no, this is what small-town life is going to be like—I'm going to hit up against this stuff a lot." She hasn't gone out on a date since.

Before I had Scott, I heard these women talking, and I thought, yeah, yeah—somehow it'll be different for me. I'll make it work. I'm a flexible, spontaneous person, I won't have to worry. Then I got a taste of reality.

When Scott was almost six months old, I had my first real date—you know, the kind where there actually appears to be interest on both sides. I invited her over for a cozy supper and video night, and figured Scott would be his usual easygoing self, napping for an hour around seven or eight and going to sleep for the night around eleven or twelve. Hell, no. Suddenly he transformed himself into Clingy Demanding Baby, not wanting me to put him down for a moment or he'd fuss. He didn't want to sleep for one moment, either. Finally, at one-thirty in the morning, he passed out on the sofa. My date lingered for another hour, probably wondering if anything was gonna happen between us. I wondered, too, but I was so tired by that point, having spent all my energy keeping the baby quiet, and I knew the nanny was coming in the morning. I just couldn't bring myself to do anything to prolong the evening. Also, frankly, I am a total wimp about making the first move. At last, she gave up and left, and I scooped the sleeping baby off the sofa and put him to bed. And realized with horror that if I am going to get any, my dates will have to go a little more like this:

"Look," I'll say brusquely, glancing at my watch after a few minutes of small talk, "I think you're cute. I don't have a lot of time to waste before the baby wakes up or the babysitter goes home. So: You in or you out? If you're in, let's get this show on the road. Kiss me. Now."

Not sure I could ever pull something like that off, but there's no telling what the specter of two decades of celibacy will do to a gal.

There are some who aren't scared of celibacy, though. "A guy would have to chase me down," says Marcy. "The only relationship I have room for is my relationship with my son." And for Marcy, it's also a question of return on emotional investment. "I'm never gonna regret the time I put into having a child," she says. "And I have often regretted the time I put into a relationship with a man."

## RELATIONSHIP SUCCESS STORIES

For single moms who really still want to find love or sex or both, it's out there and it's possible. Of the four single moms I know best (only one of whom I interviewed for this book), not one of them stayed single for long. And three of them found what appear to be happy, stable life partnerships.

That's what Jessica's looking for. "I've been dating a lot," says Jessica, mother of thirteen-month-old Ariana. "I thought having Ariana would be a deterrent for a guy, but it turns out to be the opposite. I think they feel the pressure's off." Where does she meet all these guys? Anywhere and everywhere, she says, sounding very *Sex and the City* indeed. One she met over the summer at Shelter Island, others out with friends, one was "an aging rock star" she met on a plane, another she met through her family. "My daughter goes to sleep at seven," Jessica says, "so I come home, spend time with her, and then go out again. The only conflict is, I'm up at the crack of dawn regardless, so I go out, but I have to be home by midnight." She dated one of the guys for almost six months. "He was great with the baby and all that," she says. But she hopes she can find a husband before her daughter gets much older. "The older they get, the more careful you have to be."

Liz looks like she might be on her way to a solid partnership. About a year after she and her last girlfriend broke up, she is seeing someone new, and five months into it, it's working out well, and Liz is considering starting to integrate her new girlfriend into her family more. "There's a way in which it's easier to date now," she says. "You don't have to have all these hypothetical conversations about 'Do you want kids?' The good thing about having a kid already is that people have to make a choice immediately as to whether they want that or not." It forces your dates to be more honest, she says, but it also forces you to be more honest about what you want, too. "I'm very clear now about what I want out of a relationship," she concludes. "I have two kids and they are my priority. I don't have to fight or explain it or even talk about it, it's just a fact of my life."

Some single moms think that their decision to have a baby solo will be good for their love life, and not just because the childbearing pressure is off. Maybe, they think, with a kid in the picture, they will become less attracted to the same old bad boys and more open to good guys. "I hope I'll find I'm attracted to different things," says Jamie, echoing what many other women told me. "I see myself meeting a single father somewhere."

That's what happened to Samantha, who had previously found herself attracted only to "commitmentphobes." After not even a year of single motherhood, she got involved with an old friend who became single and whom she suddenly saw in a different light. He wasn't afraid to commit, and now they have three kids—his toddler from his previous marriage, hers from her single-mom days, and a newborn they conceived together.

And though the path to single motherhood can prove too challenging for many new relationships, there are those that do weather the storm. Diana was the single mother of a two-year-old and was about to try for a sibling when she met a new man through the Internet. At first, she put her pregnancy attempts on hold. Her new guy "wasn't resistant to the idea of having kids," but since he already had two of his own from a previous marriage, he didn't necessarily feel the need for more, either. "He considered being the bio-dad" to her second child, Diana says, "but he wanted to be married and living together first, and I wasn't ready for either of those things. We weren't at that stage in the relationship."

Mindful of her advancing age, Diana ended up deciding to go forward with her plans, and started trying to conceive with anonymous-donor sperm. "I wasn't sure if he would want to stay in the relationship or not," she says. "It was a pretty low period for us." Diana didn't really talk to him about it during the insemination process. He would have wanted to be involved, she explains, but as her husband, or at least as the man sharing her home. "It was hard for him to see himself as a valued partner without those things," she says.

Diana did conceive, and the cloud lifted. "Once I was pregnant and it was a fact on the ground," she says, "then he reconciled himself to the circumstances and decided that, regardless of the circumstances, he wanted to be part of this." Her boyfriend was at her side when Diana's second baby was born a year ago, and the relationship has deepened to the point where they plan to be married this summer. Having a partner has been a massive adjustment for Diana and has changed the dynamic of her formerly single-parent family. It's been a challenge, but there have been many rewards. "He's an amazing father—he's very enthusiastic—and he's really great with my kids," Diana says. So far, happily ever after.

# Being Single
# and Pregnant

You did this to me, you bastard!" These are words that many pregnant women regard as their birthright to utter, if not sometime in the ninth month, then definitely during labor. Guess what? You won't be shouting them if you're a single mother by choice. There's no way around it—you did this to yourself.

Being pregnant is really cool—watching the amazing changes in your body and seeing your child grow inside you. But, truth be told, being alone and pregnant can really suck—although after a few months you do have a kicking little creature to keep you company. I remember cozy nights in bed alone, watching my belly dance. Many single moms by choice find pregnancy to be the hardest part of the process. "It was scary and lonely," admits Shannon, now the happy mom of a two-year-old girl. "I didn't enjoy my pregnancy as much as I hoped I would. It was depressing not to have anyone to share it with. My friends were excited for me, but it wasn't the same as having a husband. It was hard not having anyone to run to the store or rub my back." Pregnancy can be grueling, both physically and emotionally, and as a single mom by choice, there's no partner to turn to (or turn on) in a moment of frustration.

"It's harder to get sympathy," says Anne. "It's partly my own reticence, but it feels like since I made the decision to do this, then I can't really complain about it." For her, being pregnant as a single mom was harder than when she had a boyfriend. "You can't tell anyone, 'You gotta pamper me.'"

But there are definitely good points. For one thing, when you take up the entire bed, no one complains about it. "By the time I was nine months pregnant, my ankles were gigantic and I looked terrible, I really did," says Marcy, who has a two-year-old son. "I was grateful I didn't have to worry about what a guy thought of me!" Being single, you have no one to disappoint, and even better, no one to disappoint you: "I remember being in the childbirth class," Marcy reports, "and there were ten or twelve married couples. The guys looked so uncomfortable, and I was reveling in the fact that I didn't have to deal with that." And while you may not have a partner, you'll find yourself getting support from the community at large, with strangers beaming as your belly gets bigger.

Pretty much everyone agrees, though—pregnancy is a big deal, and going it alone an even bigger one. I spoke to Jenny, an artist in Brooklyn, when she was nineteen weeks pregnant. "I feel like every three or four weeks I hit another spot of realization, and I can't stop crying. Oh my God, this is so huge, I can't even wrap my head around it."

## GETTING THE GOOD NEWS

For more than a year, I was a candidate for Home Pregnancy Testers Anonymous. Every month when I was trying to conceive I vowed I wouldn't buy any home pregnancy tests; I'd wait till the more definitive blood test at my doctor's office. After all, it was only two weeks. But as the second week began, I'd be online, double-checking which was the most effective home test and when was the absolute earliest you could use it. And every month I'd cave and duck into the drugstore at least a day before the blood test. At home in the bathroom I'd stare at the one pink line (negative) and curse myself, because I knew the results were inconclusive. A positive home test would mean I was definitely pregnant, but a negative test might just mean my body hadn't yet kicked out enough of the pregnancy hormone to register on the test stick. In other words, I could still be pregnant. I was out nearly twenty dollars for nothing. I did it every month. That's fourteen times twenty dollars. Almost as bad as a Starbucks habit.

Then, in October 2005, I was scheduled for the blood test on Thursday the thirteenth. Wednesday morning dawned and I couldn't stand it anymore. I had an extra test lying around from a two-pack (I had managed to control myself the month before and only use one of them). I used it, splashing it too much. Almost immediately there was a Rorschach pattern of pink; pink was oozing everywhere, illegible. What the?! Was this two lines at last? Or was this just a mistake, with excessive urination causing the thing to go kerflooey? Dammit, was I pregnant or did I screw up the test? It was pouring rain and I was nervous as anything. I ran through the rain to the drugstore and bought two different kinds of tests: a two-pack of the regular kind and an idiotproof one that actually said "pregnant" if you were pregnant. I brought them back and turned my bathroom into a sitcom cliché, pregnancy tests everywhere. I tried one, paced around my bedroom, and then went back to the sink. Double line. No way. Tried another. Double line. Tried the third. Pregnant. Pregnant. Pregnant!

So if you're single, whom do you race to with the good news? My answer was, everybody! Well, at least my family and all my close friends. It would have been almost impossible not to, since everyone close to me knew I'd been trying for so long, and they always asked how it was going. Besides, I didn't feel the need to keep early pregnancy a secret in case of miscarriage—for me, having friends know what was going on would make it easier to cope if I lost the baby, not harder. Married couples often keep pregnancy to themselves for the first trimester, in case of miscarriage and maybe also so they can have a secret to share. But most single moms by choice tell their close friends, like I did. Many hold off on telling their families, though, if they haven't told them of their single motherhood plans and fear judgment or negativity.

## EASY PREGNANCIES: THEY DO EXIST!

I heard all sorts of dire warnings about pregnancy from my friend Rose, who'd had a baby, and my friend Sally, whose many sisters had about one hundred babies among them, or so Sally—a bit of a storyteller—made it sound. The doom-and-gloom sisters, I called them behind their backs. When I got bronchitis at about six weeks pregnant and felt completely exhausted, as I always do with bronchitis, Rose assured me, "Oh, no, it's not the bronchitis, it's pregnancy, and lemme tell you, it's gonna get worse from here on out." She'd then list all the terrible things I could expect for sure, starting with heartburn (never had it) and ending with not being able to walk without searing pubic-bone pain (didn't happen). Where Rose left off, Sally started in, with the authority of one who has seen a thousand pregnancies, all of them hard. "Shut *up*!" I'd tell them. I knew there were all sorts of horrible things that could happen. But my sister and my mom had easy pregnancies. Maybe I would, too.

The fact is, terrible pregnancies happen, but easy ones do, too. A number of the women I interviewed were lucky enough to have the latter kind. "From everything I've heard, I've had the easiest pregnancy ever," says Nina, who was doing standup comedy almost to her eighth month, when standing for so long got a little tiresome. "I've had some heartburn, but that's about it."

Lisa S. not only had an "incredibly easy" pregnancy and delivery, but she says between her thirteen-year-old daughter and her mom, she never felt alone. Single moms with families who live close by often have this important level of support. Liz's parents didn't live close, but "my aunt and uncle came with me to all my appointments," she says. Then, when she had her twins on Thanksgiving Day, it was a family holiday. "My aunt and uncle, my mom, my stepfather, everybody was at the hospital."

"I had an easy, great pregnancy," recalls Jessica, who lives in Manhattan. "This is one of the great things about living in New York. There isn't a lot of isolation here. Even the little things like getting your coffee, your routine, is social." Jessica frequented the diner and the bakery: "I was hooked on grilled cheese and tomato and cupcakes," she says. "Everybody was really nice to us. I have a poodle, so I was the pregnant lady with the poodle." She made up for any loneliness by trying to pamper herself. "I got in the bathtub every morning, and that was very fun for me. My baby didn't kick very much—she was just happy floating in there—but I'd get in the bathtub and I could see her little heartbeat." So baths were a special time for Jessica bonding with her baby. "Turns out I was looking at *my* heartbeat," Jessica discovered later, and laughs. "Well, you know what, it worked for me at the time!" Normally fashionable, Jessica took care not to devolve into a schlub in sweatpants. "I was always dressed. I wanted to feel good," she says. "My doctor said, 'You're so *Sex and the City*, Jessica—you've got the shoes, you've got the whole bit.'"

"I loved being pregnant," says Elisa. "As crazy as it sounds, I loved being enormous. Walking around in my yoga pants with my big belly hanging out. I loved that my body image was no longer an issue but an empowering experience. I loved being able to balance things on my belly. I just had a lot of fun with it."

Elisa's single-mother-by-choice independence got away from her a little, though. "I moved when I was eight months pregnant and I thought I could pack everything up myself, and I ended up breaking my foot. It was really almost comical. The foot had been fractured before, and the hospital ended up keeping me there longer than usual because they thought it might have something to do with domestic violence." The hospital didn't really buy her story of packing up for a move on her own. Surely, a pregnant woman would have help. "I said no, believe me, the only one beating me up is me." She now realizes she took self-sufficiency way, way too far (for more on that, see Chapter 10). "There's some crazy independent part of me that's proud I was able to put together the crib at eight months pregnant," she says. "You know what, get someone to help you, girlfriend!"

As it turned out, I had an easy pregnancy, too, with very little to complain about. No morning sickness, no heartburn, not much fatigue. The worst ongoing problem was the painful spider veins that appeared on my left calf at about three months and made it so I had to wear grandma medical support stockings for half a year (tip: they now make 'em in black—equally uncomfortable, but you can pretend they're just saucy thigh-highs), including on the beach (now, that was a great look). I was able to be extremely active till I delivered, with the exception of two bouts of bronchitis, a few weeks of modified bed rest due to bleeding, and a couple days in the hospital with kidney stones (more on that later). My pregnancy, by and large, was problem free. But believe me, even if you have plenty to complain about, *no one wants to hear it.* ("I think every single mom should have a designated friend that they can just bitch to anytime day or night," says Anne, engaging in a little wishful thinking.) That's the beauty of the husband for most pregnant women. You can in fact guilt him into listening to you whine, since it could be argued that he got you in this predicament. He—or your female partner and coparent, if that's your setup—may actually even *want* to listen. But alas for us single moms by choice. Maybe we can get our parents or best friends to listen occasionally. But in general, it's gotta be stiff upper lip. (That's where online support groups can come in handy.)

Yet even a relatively problem-free pregnancy has its challenges, and I did break down once. It was during my second bad bout of bronchitis. I was five months pregnant, and it was my fourth trip up my three flights of stairs with my elderly (read: bladder-impaired) dog, in from the freezing cold, sick as, well, a dog, this time carrying heavy bags of groceries filled with cans of chicken soup since I was out of food. I felt beyond terrible and collapsed in a blubbering heap toward the top of the stairs. Then (this was a big step for me), instead of just sucking it up as usual, I called my mom. She must have been so freaked out! I don't think I'd ever, *ever* done something like that to her before. I'd always been the dutiful oldest daughter, keeping my emotions under tight control. Before I knew it, she was offering to drive the six hours from Richmond to Brooklyn to pick up my dog and bring him home to her house. My mom rocks.

There were some dark times in my pregnancy, though, that transcended routine illness or garden-variety loneliness. Toward the end of my first trimester I started bleeding, just the way I had when I miscarried before. The bleeding came pretty heavily, then backed off, then heavier again, then went on for almost a month. Turns out my placenta was lying low, a fairly common thing. I was "probably" not miscarrying again, the doctors said, and it would "probably" resolve itself. It did, and no harm done. But, boy, I really could have used a partner to help comfort and distract me.

Then, in my sixth and seventh months, I had three episodes of severe abdominal pain, apparently related to dehydration (despite drinking water like a fiend, I became dehydrated at the drop of a hat). The first was terrifying, because I was vacationing on a remote island, far from good medical care, but it was short-lived and my sister was with me. The second time I was in New York, alone, and ended up in the hospital for half the night, but all in all it wasn't too bad. The third time was the worst, with pain worse than labor, the nurses told me (my face got scraped up from writhing in pain against the rough hospital sheets). I was in agony for ten hours until they gave me morphine. They think it was probably a kidney stone. My crazy friend Joni—a platinum-haired, jackbooted East Village punk-rock chick (and Ph.D. candidate) with the thickest broad-from–Staten Island accent you ever heard—happened to have been visiting when this happened. Joni took me to the hospital and stayed with me all night, bless her, feeding me crushed ice, cracking jokes, making fun of me to distract me from the pain— and making sure the nurses did their job. You don't mess around with Joni.

She says she's got friends who'll break kneecaps, though something in her manner tells you that without her even having to mention it.

I was terrified only when she went out for a burger and I had a long wave of pain so severe that I thought it would make me lose consciousness and no one was going to know because the curtains to my triage cubicle were drawn. But the next morning the pain had subsided, thanks to the morphine, and Joni went home. I called a handful of friends I thought might have flexible schedules. It wasn't convenient for any of them to stay with me that day. I thought that would probably be OK, and I didn't want to put anyone out too much. Turns out it really wasn't OK at all. I needed a helper and advocate and I suffered quite a bit as a result of not having one. It was the kind of situation where if I'd had a partner, she would have stayed with me, no question. But I didn't. It made me realize that, as a single mother, I was going to have two choices in times of need: rely heavily on friends, something I was not initially comfortable with, or suffer. And next time, the person to suffer because of my reluctance to ask for help might not be me—it might be my child.

## HARD PREGNANCY: A POSSIBILITY TO BE PREPARED FOR

Despite the bouts of illness, I'd describe my pregnancy as an exceptionally easy one. I was healthy, active, and, for the most part, joyful, out swing dancing six hours before my water broke. Not everyone's so lucky. Cheri has had high blood pressure since her late twenties, and that started to cause complications toward the end of her pregnancy. They told her to cut back her activity as much as possible. That was hard. "Here I am, a single woman, trying to get the nursery ready, so I was pushing myself a lot."

Amanda had even more complications. When she was just into her second trimester of pregnancy as a single-mom-to-be, Amanda was admitted to the hospital with serious high blood pressure. Her nose was bleeding—they explained, "Your blood pressure is so high the blood wants to come out however it can." The young intern on duty tried to figure out what was going on. "At one point I looked out and he was standing in the hall, kind of banging his head against the wall," Amanda says. "I thought, This is not good."

Amanda turned out to have a rare and life-threatening condition called

HELLP syndrome, which involves high blood pressure and low platelets. "The good news is your liver is working," they told her. "The bad news is you have no platelets, so you might bleed to death." They were able to get her blood pressure under control, but she stayed in the hospital for weeks, her health on an alarming roller-coaster ride. "Every few days there was talk of going home," Amanda says. "I finally told the doctor they had to stop saying that, because every time you mention it, some other organ ceases functioning." They put her on an IV and wouldn't let her eat for ten days in case of surgery, but then a hospital staffer mentioned that it would be hard to get a surgeon to perform an emergency C-section because she'd bleed out.

It was terrifying. Amanda happened to have a cousin who was a neonatal intensive-care nurse, and two best friends, one who was an emergency-room nurse and the other an internal-medicine doctor, so that helped a lot. She took it in stride, in part because there wasn't another option. "When the choice is, if you don't do this, the baby's going to die, what are you going to do?" Amanda says. "The fear thing—I just tried not to think about it." Her parents came to stay and were at the hospital with her every day. "My friends and family put themselves on a schedule," she says. And Amanda eventually settled into the hospital routine.

Amy didn't end up in the hospital, but had a difficult pregnancy for other reasons. "I had been a very active, fit runner, biker, and swimmer," Amy says, "then the morning sickness hit and I basically couldn't get off the couch. I had terrible back pain; it hurt terribly to walk. I was miserable the entire time, from week six until I went into labor. There was not one day that I felt normal, and I'm not exaggerating." Worst of all, she was alone and did not know how to reach out for support. Amy became clinically depressed, but her doctors, in addition to being judgmental and nonsupportive about her single-mom status, refused to take her depression seriously. "Every month that I went for my checkup, I cried and asked for antidepressants and the doctors said no." This is where a little extra advance research or a trip to a psychiatrist might have helped Amy—there are antidepressants that are approved for use in pregnancy if necessary, and certainly no pregnant woman should reach that level of depression without some sort of support, whether pharmacological or emotional or both. But when you're having problems, it can be hard to seek help. "I did think about switching obstetricians, but I was so exhausted and felt like crap, and to take the energy to be switching doctors, it was just too much." But Amy wishes she had considered how important a supportive ob-gyn was going to be, and she also wishes she had known about online support groups. "I now know how to just get on e-mail and find ten pregnant women who are just a car ride away. Even e-mail is support, and you don't have to know them. You can feel comfort from a stranger. You have to create a support network, but when I was pregnant I didn't know what that meant."

For Charlene, as for some other single moms by choice I spoke to, pregnancy actually brought out some problems with the support network she already had. She realized it often went only one way. "When you choose to have a family at this age [Charlene was forty-two] and you've been single for a while," Charlene explains, "there are things that other people count on you to do." As the friend who's single and always available, you may be crucial to other people's support systems, and by having a child you end up having much less to give, because you're necessarily focusing on your baby and yourself. That transition won't always be welcome for those around you who have come to depend on you. For Charlene, it was most evident during her pregnancy, which was a difficult one, with constant morning sickness—"I threw up for eight and a half months till my eyeballs ruptured and my nose bled"—stress incontinence, and gestational diabetes. "My work needed me to be a forty-two-year-old bitch project manager; they did not want this sick pregnant lady," Charlene says. "My family needed me to be the eldest daughter who takes care of everything. And my friends were used to me being the caretaker, the mom." Charlene found herself much more alone than she had anticipated.

## LONELINESS

Most of the women I talked to said they weren't lonely during their pregnancies. I'm not sure I'm buying it. I think loneliness and isolation have got to be the biggest issues for pregnant single women. When you're pregnant and single, there are countless times you're reminded that everyone else has a partner. There you are, the only single woman on the hospital tour, as your fellow tourists file past the birthing rooms in pairs, all holding hands, the husbands trying to outdo each other in solicitousness toward their wives. There you are again, the only single woman in the waiting room for special prenatal testing, the husbands looking properly concerned or distracting their wives with conversation. Once again, there's you—the only single woman in childbirth class. Who are these superhuman women who don't feel lonely? In any case, I'm not one of them. I was terribly lonely at times. Also, during my pregnancy, many of my usual social invitations dried up. Mainly it was a question of happenstance—friends becoming mired in new relationships and new jobs or both; I think I also may have gone from A list to B list with some people after a breakup the year before (my ex was their good friend, too). Then one good friend was out of town for four months. Whatever the reason, I found myself much more alone than I had anticipated—and I had anticipated being alone.

The worst was when I was sick for weeks with bronchitis, feeling crummy and forced to spend hours on the sofa with nothing to think about but poor, poor me, romantic dreams of shared parenthood dashed, pregnant and all alone, no one to whine to, no one to fix me soup, no one to walk the dog, no one to cuddle with, no one who gave a shit about feeling the baby kick, no one, no one, no one.

I can joke about it now, and really, bronchitis aside, as someone who could successfully get pregnant at forty-two and who could afford to sit and feel sorry for herself while watching digital cable on a luxurious velvet-covered Crate & Barrel couch, my real-world pathos quotient was pretty darned low. But it felt quite painful at the time. I had wanted so badly to be doing this with a partner.

If I'd had a regular office job, daily interactions with my colleagues might have taken up some of the social slack. Instead, I leaned on a community of acquaintances and near strangers (and sometimes total strangers), and the truth is, between moments of dire loneliness every week or two, for the most part I felt happy, independent, and not lonely at all. I went to dance classes every Tuesday, and took part in two different dance performances while I was pregnant (the last performance I was six months pregnant and leading in a bouncy Charleston number). I went out dancing again every Thursday night, and sometimes again on Saturday. I went to the gym at least twice a week, my writer's group met every Wednesday, prenatal yoga was Saturday afternoon, and every morning I'd stop by the same café while walking my dog.

Not only did this give me a lot of regular socializing, but slowly, as I got more pregnant, I became more of an oddity and people started to sort of adopt me as a mascot, perhaps because I wasn't lying on the sofa like normal pregnant ladies. As That Pregnant Lady, I was greeted with special warmth, and people would comment on my size and ask how I was feeling, and even ask to touch my belly, which, since no one was doing it at home, I quite welcomed. I became pals with the kindly cleaning woman at the gym and the pair of pert blond twentysomethings who told me I was an inspiration. Occasionally some muscle-bound guy would give me the thumbs-up. Even the cashiers at my neighborhood grocery and retired guys who hung out at the café became part of my support system. In fact, when I went back to my Thursday night dance after the baby was born and stopped by the convenience store for my usual late-night bottle of water and Luna bar, the cashier there was beaming, wanting to know all about Scott, insisting I bring him by one night, practically ready to give me a baby present. This is a guy who saw me for thirty seconds once a week as I made a three-dollar purchase.

Yes, during my pregnancy I literally soaked up support wherever I found it. Even if your friends aren't wildly interested, there are plenty of people out there who get excited about pregnancy and babies. I know many pregnant women find such attention intrusive, even enraging. But as a single pregnant woman with no one fussing over me at home, that community of interest and support meant a lot to me. I was blessed with an easy pregnancy and the ability to stay physically active, though in my last trimester I often felt exhausted and uncomfortable. If I'd had a partner I am certain I would have spent most nights curled up on the couch, angling for a back rub. But my couch was a lonely place to be, so I dragged myself out and it almost always made me feel better. Most of my scheduled social activities were physical ones, but they could just have well been knitting classes or a book group. In any case, I'd recommend creating such consistent community for yourself, because there are definitely times when being pregnant and single is gonna suck, and your friends may not always be right there.

The Saturday before Scott was born, I went to prenatal yoga and then stopped by the farmers' market for some geraniums. I then waddled home in my tank top, yoga pants, and medical support stockings, all 215 unwashed, sweaty pounds of me schlepping two big plastic bags full of flowerpots. As I concentrated on trying to ignore the giant baby head that hammered my bladder with every step, an older woman's voice shouted down to me from a third-floor balcony: "YOU LOOK BEAUTIFUL!" Now, much as I'd like to think so, I doubt that was true. Certainly I did not possess a radiance that would cause people to shout from the rooftops. She was just giving me a "Right on, sistah!" But it made my day. I practically floated home on pink geranium blossoms. I don't know who she was, but bless her! I'll never forget her.

Julie says she was lonely, too. She kept herself busy and social during her pregnancy, but "when I was sleeping alone at night and uncomfortable, or home alone feeling tired on the couch, I felt very lonely," she says. "I wanted to be sharing it with a partner, so part of being pregnant was kind of grieving the fact that here I was doing it alone."

Jenny, who was in her second trimester of pregnancy when I spoke to her, admits to loneliness as well. "I miss having someone to accompany me, going through this insanely miraculous process," she says. "My girlfriends with children are the biggest rocks for me." Her married friends also help her keep her single-mom loneliness in perspective. "My friends with husbands are like, the men have no idea and we're basically going through it alone," Jenny says. She was on the phone with one friend who's a mom, talking about the experience of having a kid. The friend said, "Hold on," and then Jenny waited as she heard the friend walk up the stairs and shut her bedroom door to keep her husband from hearing what she was about to say and getting hurt by it.

"Imagine how much you would love the person you fall in love with," her friend whispered. "You're going to love your child a thousand times more."

Jenny says she tries to ward off disappointment by not expecting support from those who don't have it to give, by accepting help from those who offer. "I've had people say, 'Anytime you need something just call me,' and those are the people I call. Still, going through a pregnancy as a single mom by choice can be a breathtakingly lonely experience. Jenny describes making the decision about whether or not to have an amniocentesis as one of her lonelier moments. The amnio is a test that can tell you if the baby has certain chromosomal abnormalities, like Down syndrome. But the test carries a slight risk of causing a miscarriage. Then if there are abnormalities, you are faced with the decision of whether or not to terminate the pregnancy, which by that time is into the second trimester. For Jenny, the stressful part was making the decision to get the test in the first place. "It was a really hard decision to make, I had to make it on my own, and it was just one of many huge decisions I was going to have to make on my own. I was crying for days." She ended up deciding to have the amnio, and she felt good about it. Still, the experience really highlighted for her how alone a single mom can be sometimes.

For me, the amniocentesis was the scariest point in my pregnancy. I wanted the information, but I had no idea what I would decide if my baby had Down syndrome. While I am pro-choice, I wasn't sure I could have an abortion unless the problem were much more severe than Down's. I knew I was scared, and I knew I was working not to let my fear obsess me. In fact, my attempts at emotional self-control were working beautifully. I had been really unbelievably calm since the test was taken; it almost seemed to me like I wasn't worried at all. I started to believe my own "laid-back" hype. I didn't realize just how scared I was until my doctor's head nurse called me on my cell phone with the results one Friday afternoon, sooner than expected. She caught me at the local mail-services shop, trying to send a fax. "Did you want to know the sex?" she asked. "Yes," I said. "You're having a baby boy. He's totally healthy." I thanked her and immediately burst into tears. Some of the other patrons were concerned and asked me if I was OK. "Yes!" I said, sobbing so hard I could barely be understood, and I tried to explain the news, that I had just found out I was having a healthy boy. "Congratulations!" everyone said, and then everyone looked uncomfortable as I sobbed "Thanks!" and tried to give them a cheery smile, tears running down my blotchy cheeks. "Are you upset because it's not a girl?" one of them asked, concerned, after an awkward silence. "No!" I sobbed, unable to stop. "I'm just so happy it's healthy!" I could not stop crying for the rest of the day, I was so grateful and relieved. Someone suggested it was pregnancy hormones. Could have been, but I wasn't particularly moody during my pregnancy. I think it was more the enormity of the issue, and my relief at having dodged making a decision that would have been unbearably hard for me, either way.

Worse than simply being alone, though, is enlisting the help of someone who doesn't come through. Not having your spouse potentially disappoint you is a plus to single pregnancy. But it's not only spouses that can let us down. One of the lonelier times for me was right before I had my twenty-week fetal ultrasound. That's the one you hear about the most and see on TV, where moms- and dads-to-be are oohing and aahing over the little fingers and toes and looking to see if they can tell the sex, if they haven't been tipped off earlier by the chromosomes (aka the amniocentesis). I anticipated that I would go to that appointment alone, and I was OK with it. I was just looking forward to seeing my baby. But then months beforehand, a friend asked if she could join me. She really, really wanted to see, she said. I was happy and excited to have her company and enthusiasm, and I recategorized the experience in my mind as one of the few things I would *not* be doing alone. I was so happy about that. Then, the day before the appointment, my friend called. "Sorry, I can't make it. The cable guys didn't come today, so I have to reschedule for tomorrow." I was angry and upset, and told her how much I had been counting on her to accompany me. She then agreed to reschedule the cable appointment again and join me after all. The morning of the appointment, I got another call. "My cat is sick, I can't leave him." I had to go to the ultrasound alone. On the way to the hospital I was crying, feeling desperately lonely, dreading being in that waiting room again with all the married couples—but I was also furious, not just at my friend but at myself, because I knew my negative feelings were all about my expectations. If my friend hadn't asked to join me, I never would have expected company, and instead of feeling sad and alone going to this momentous appointment, I would have felt only excitement and happiness.

Then again, at the end of my pregnancy, except for the no-sex thing, which, like the baby's head on my bladder, just became more painful with each passing day, I started to see how it might be a blessing to be single. Maybe someone would have wanted to have sex with me, but I cannot imagine who would have been able to put up with sleeping with me. It was toss, turn, toss, turn, all night long. The last month I was often up every hour on the hour, either because I had to pee again or because my hip bones hurt so much I couldn't bear it. I was stoic about it, mainly because there wasn't anyone to complain to. But I imagine I would have been whining constantly if I'd had a captive listening audience, and unless I was domestically partnered with Mother Teresa herself, there probably would have been some major fights.

Though I am officially suspicious of many of the single moms I spoke to who claim their pregnancies were not lonely, there's at least one of them whose story I believe. Alice says she really enjoyed her pregnancy and never felt alone. That's probably because she wasn't—her mom had moved in with her, her coworkers were supportive, and she had a very active, social after-work life. "I played tennis and I refereed rugby and I played softball well into my seventh month," she says, "and I was running into my last month." May every single mom's pregnancy be like that!

## WHO'S YOUR LABOR COACH?

I had always dreamed that when I had a baby, my partner would be there, cheering me on, showering me with kisses, and rubbing whatever part of me needed to be rubbed. Candles would be lit, yadda yadda yadda. Once I embarked on my solo pregnancy, I knew this wouldn't be the case, but I still couldn't give up the dream or come up with a replacement scenario that felt right. Some of the friends I'd known the longest and felt the most comfortable with lived out of state. Ditto with my family. And I was nervous about the extreme nakedness. I'm comfortable with a certain amount of flesh showing, mind you. When I was about six weeks pregnant, I'd performed in a crazy dance number in which the costume was a miniskirt that at one point came off momentarily (as part of the choreography), leaving all of us standing in our underwear in front of three hundred people. That exposure was supposed to last about two seconds. But I had a wardrobe malfunction à la Janet Jackson—my miniskirt wouldn't go back on as planned and I had to finish out the number with the bottom half of my costume trailing behind me like so much toilet paper. I was embarrassed to think of what my thighs must look like, but I went on with the show, occasionally working the skirt like a feather boa to make the mistake look like part of the production. The crowd stomped and cheered and gave us a standing ovation. I was fine with that. But total nakedness? I've always been super shy in that regard. I won't skinny-dip unless it's a dark, dark night. I don't go topless on beaches in Europe. When I went to a nude beach with friends once, I wore a swimsuit. So the idea of being naked, spread-legged, and screaming in front of some random friend? I could not even imagine it. I think even into the eighth month I was hoping for the love of my life to suddenly materialize, mainly so I didn't have to deal with finding a friend to be with me for the birth.

It wasn't just about nakedness, of course. I had let go of my dream of having a child with a partner enough to actually get pregnant alone, enough to make a will and name guardians, enough to be ready to raise a child by myself. But I was still holding on tight to part of the dream—the part where, in the intense pain, utter vulnerability, and once-in-a-lifetime beauty of childbirth, I would have at my side someone who loved me, loved the child, and for whom the experience would be as intimate and profound as it would be for me.

Yeah, well, no dice. When you're a single mom by choice, your birthing partners won't necessarily be who you would have chosen. You just have to suck it up, make a choice, and know that it will be a beautiful experience regardless. "There just aren't a lot of people who you really want to see you in that situation," says Nina, who was a month from delivery when I spoke to her. She ended up picking a friend she was really "in synch" with, she says, who was very grounded and had taken some massage classes, and she was hopeful it would go well.

Julie had her sister there as her labor-support person, but she also had Paul, her coparent/sperm donor. Julie had a natural childbirth in a birthing center, so there she was, naked and moaning, being supported by her sister and by Paul, someone she saw as something closer to a business partner. It was uncomfortable to say the least. All she could do was try to block it out.

Jocelyn didn't have the perfect labor-support person in mind so she ended up with a tag team, her sister and her friend Stephanie. "My sister is notoriously nonempathetic to pain and suffering," Jocelyn says, "but she wanted to be there, she was enthusiastic, and she's reliable. Stephanie's notoriously late and flaky, but very empathetic. It worked out perfectly to have both of them. As it turned out, I was in labor for four days. I think they were both glad there were two of them."

For Jessica, the issue was finding someone she could really count on to be there for her in labor. "People have their own lives," she says. She had a lot of friends volunteer, but she didn't feel secure about anyone. "People have really good intentions, but . . . I wasn't comfortable that they'd come through." In fact, the friend who went to the hospital with her left to walk Jessica's dog and didn't turn up until after the baby was born. She'd run into Jessica's brother and they'd been hanging out at the corner bar. "I wasn't going to get into a fight with anybody," Jessica says. "I was fine, the baby was fine." Fortunately, Jessica had hired a doula, which is a birth assistant whose focus is helping the mother through the process. "No one else would rub your back for eight hours straight," says Jessica. "It was great."

Tauz, who when I spoke to her was four months pregnant "and so loving it," has no worries about her birth attendants. During her pregnancy there have been lonely moments—"When certain things are changing about my body or if I hear the baby's heartbeat, I find myself wishing I had someone

to share that with"—but her home birth looks like it will be a group celebration. She has her best friend lined up as her main source of support. "We
talked about how difficult single motherhood might be and she always promised me that if I was going to do it, she'd be there for me. So I said I was ready
to do it, and she said, 'I'm ready to support you.'" But in addition, another
good friend—a massage therapist and Reiki master—will be visiting from
Washington State, and she'll also have a midwife.

Many of the single moms I spoke to hired a doula to be there with them,
in addition to family or friends. Doulas don't deliver the baby, but they have
a bag of tricks to help ease the pain of labor, and they'll rub your back (for
hours, as Jessica discovered) and feed you ice chips and do most of what your
dream partner would be doing. They'll come to your house when you're in
active labor and accompany you to the hospital when it's time. In fact, many
married or partnered women hire doulas to take the pressure off
their partners and to make sure someone who knows what they are doing
is there for them. For a single woman who can afford it, it can really make
a difference.

Toward the end of my pregnancy, my friends Susanna and Melodie offered
to be my labor coaches. I still wasn't at all comfortable with the idea, but I
was touched by their generosity and they seemed genuinely excited about it.
I'd hired a doula and felt very comfortable with her, but I finally decided that
it was ridiculous to only have hired professionals attending the birth. Susanna and Melodie knew me and cared about me, and I needed to just get
over my pathological modesty and my white-knuckled grip on an inaccessi-
ble romantic dream. It was decided. They had Melodie's mom on standby to
take their one-year-old daughter, and I spent the rest of my pregnancy trying to get used to the idea of sharing the experience—my plan was to have
a drug-free birth in the hospital's gorgeous natural birthing center, complete
with Jacuzzi—with them. We made a date for a Friday night, my due date,
to really talk it over, maybe practice some massage. I had Scott on Thursday, the day before.

There are some people, whether through luck or temperament or both,
who just don't need much help. "Since I'm in the military," says Marcy, "and
my family is far away, I didn't have much of a support system during my
pregnancy and still don't today. I called a coworker to drive me to the hospital and hired a doula for my labor, mainly because so many people told me
I absolutely could not go to the hospital and have a baby alone. In the end,

I would have done fine without her, and been seven hundred and fifty dollars richer, as the nurses were much more my style than the doula."

If you end up with a birth plan that isn't ideal, don't worry about it. Births tend not to go exactly the way you dreamed they would anyway. Mine certainly didn't. Ultimately, I'd say that for me what I heard many times was true, despite all the romantic notions I had in advance. Anne, who had two babies, said it during our interview: "When you're actually in the process of having the baby, you don't really care."

## AT LAST: THE BABY SHOWER!

There's one thing a single-mom-to-be definitely does not need to miss out on and that's the baby shower! True, one woman I spoke to never had one, because her best friend was busy freaking out about the pregnancy and what it meant for her own childbearing plans. But I learned something about celebrations one year in college when my normally attentive friends missed my subtle hints about my twenty-first birthday coming up: If you want something celebrated, don't be subtle! So much as I didn't prefer to do it that way, I was ready to strong-arm a friend into being at least the nominal hostess of my shower. If push came to shove, I figured, I could get my friend Julie to do it, since I'd cohosted her shower (and provided little plastic babies frozen into the ice cubes for the punch, a macabre touch I couldn't resist when I saw the freaky babies in the party store, and which Julie may not have forgiven me for).

I needn't have worried. My friends Melodie and Susanna, fairy godmothers of my late pregnancy, offered to throw the party at their house, and they enlisted a few more friends as cohostesses. Rose was in charge of games; Maryellen, the wine; my friends Karen and Amy, who were driving down from Rhode Island with their son Pascal, ended up in charge of paper goods; and Carolyn ordered up a huge cake. My pregnancy may have been lonely at times, but the shower was packed with friends and family, eating and drinking and ducking under decorative old-fashioned clotheslines holding onesies and tiny socks. Melodie had gone all Martha Stewart on us, arranging tulips in sippy cups and preparing an elaborate springtime feast complete with poached salmon. We played Name That Baby—people had brought in their baby pictures—and guests added ideas to my baby-name wall of white butcher paper that had been started at my housewarming party earlier that spring (Sassafras. Mercutio. Balthazar. Haasan Mohammed Ali. Somehow, none of them stuck). Rose handed out the funny quiz she'd crafted, with specialized single-mom questions like "If you add Louise's height to the height of her anonymous donor, how tall would you be?" (12'5") and "What is a liquid nitrogen tank used for?" (option C—incorrect—was "To chill the speculum before insertion during an office examination") and regular questions like "The water (amniotic fluid) surrounding the baby is . . ." (correct answer—baby pee).

Scott and I hauled in a lot of loot—cute outfits, stuffed animals, toys, books, baby towels, even a hand-me-down three-hundred-dollar electric breast pump—but more than anything it was a big public celebration of Scott's impending birth. I felt loved and taken care of. At the end of a long, often lonely winter of pregnancy, the spring shower lifted my spirits and got me primed for the big event. Somehow, those insanely small socks, more than anything, made it all start to seem very real—there's a baby in there!

# And Baby Makes Two

*Surviving the First Year*

**B**aby Scott's entrance started at about five in the morning on June 21, six hours after I'd left my usual Tuesday night swing dance and two days before his due date. I was sleeping terribly, as was usual in my last couple months of pregnancy, then I felt an extreme movement, as if the baby had flipped himself back into breech (wrong side up) position. Moments later, my water broke spectacularly, just like on TV, even though I'd heard it rarely happens that way. I'd had a false alarm once, but it was unmistakable this time. We were off!

Just try to go back to sleep after that. My out-box shows I sent an e-mail reply to an old colleague at 5:18 a.m. I forced myself back to bed but gave up after a couple more hours of fitful slumber. At nine o'clock I called my doctor, my mother, my doula, my labor-coach friends, then spent the day trying to tie up loose ends, waiting for contractions to start. They didn't. I hopped up and down, I danced around, I took castor oil, I did everything I could think of. I'd had my heart set on delivering in the hospital's cozy natural birthing center, which was on a separate floor and had totally different rules from regular labor and delivery—it would be pretty close to a home birth. But I knew if they had to use drugs to induce my labor, I'd have to be in a regular hospital room and have the highly medicalized birth I'd been trying to avoid. I hopped harder. Afternoon found me walking briskly in the park, another one of my unsuccessful attempts to bring on contractions, conducting a scheduled business meeting by cell phone. By that time my labor coaches Melodie and Susanna had come over and were trailing behind me, ready to help me if I should suddenly collapse and give birth in the bushes.

"Uh, are you *sure* you don't want to reschedule?" my business associate kept asking. The fact that I might go into labor any second was freaking her out. I figured I wasn't in pain, could use something to do, and it was the last time I wouldn't have a baby on my hands, so why not go on with the meeting?

The doctor told me if I wasn't in labor by nine o'clock that night I had to go into the hospital to be induced. By eight o'clock, the Indian takeout (spicy food, another home remedy for inducing labor) had arrived and my friend Sally had dropped by. Though I had always dreamed of a quiet, intimate birth with just my partner at my side, this single-mom birth experience was turning into a party—a fun one at that.

At nine o'clock, still not in labor, I started running nervously around my apartment trying to figure out what else to put in my bag while Melodie and Susanna cleaned up the Indian food and Sally put together a speaker system I'd bought for my iPod so I could have music during labor. My old friends Melissa and Amanda showed up in a borrowed SUV and we all piled in and headed for the hospital. I had expected an excruciating backseat ride in the throes of labor, bumping over New York City potholes; instead I sat in the front seat of a car full of friends and we laughed all the way there.

By the time we got to the hospital it was eleven o'clock and Mom had just arrived from Maine. The party continued with a brief Girl Scout–style sleepover in the hospital room—me in the bed, Mom on the pullout chair, Melodie and Susanna on hospital blankets on the floor. At five in the morning they started the IV drip of Pitocin, the drug used to induce labor, and by noon I'd been in intense contractions for a few hours. I cranked up the music, a mix of hip-hop and jazz, and when the pain hit I leaned over, holding on to the bed, swaying to the music while Jada the doula, who'd arrived around nine o'clock, rubbed my lower back. It felt like I was in a groove. My doctor's hip young Latina partner came in when the iPod was playing "Don't Go There" by rapper 24K: "Oh, no, wait a minute, don't go there 'cause I ain't wit it. . . . I aint yo' ho', don't play me like no ho!"

"Good song for delivering a boy," the doctor joked, then admonished my belly: "You treat your mama right!" Labor hurt like a mother, but so far it was also pretty fun.

By twelve-thirty it started falling apart. First the nurse kept coming in to fuss with me and readjust the fetal monitor that was strapped to my belly, because every time I got into a comfortable position for dealing with contractions, the monitor slipped and lost the baby's heartbeat. (Fetal monitors are designed for women lying flat on their backs.) Then the doctor came in and told me I hadn't progressed at all. I was exhausted after being up for a day and a half and I'd just endured hours of pretty bad pain—Pitocin causes much-harder-than-normal contractions. I had thought I was pretty close to having a baby, but the doctor said I wasn't even in active labor yet. My mom said I looked like I'd been socked in the stomach. I couldn't take fighting the system and the fetal monitor anymore—more than just painful, it was intensely irritating to have to hold still for the machine. So I decided on the epidural, and my birth experience became officially just exactly the way I hadn't wanted it: in an antiseptic hospital room, hooked up to a million machines, all drugged up. Though a numbed-out, medicalized delivery is certainly more civilized and a lot less painful. There was none of the screaming nakedness I'd been so stressed out about sharing with my friends.

In fact, my delivery was so civilized, it was timed for right after my doctor finished her regular office hours. She arrived at six o'clock and twenty minutes later she told me it was time to push—as fast as I could, because it looked like the baby might be in distress. Push with what? I couldn't feel a thing below my waist. I summoned up the memory of my abs and got to work. In the middle of a contraction, Lucinda Williams came on the iPod, singing "He Never Got Enough Love," a song about an abandoned and abused boy.

"His mama ran off when he was just a kid," she started to croon.

"Oh, no!" I panted. Wait a minute, don't go there 'cuz I ain't wit it. "Skip this one. No Lucinda during delivery!"

A half hour later, we were down to the last few pushes, with the nurse timing contractions, the doctor preparing to catch, Susanna and Melodie helping to hold back my legs, and Jada, who couldn't get near me for all the others, snapping photographs. Mom sat discreetly over by the window. I wanted to watch what was happening, but when the rolling full-length mirror arrived and was adjusted right, I stared in horror at the scene, blood red with ugly orange highlights from the Betadine. "It looks like a Georgia

O'Keeffe psychedelic nightmare!" I said. And way, *way* more like a cow giving birth than I was comfortable with. Despite the gore, it was amazing to watch Scott make his entrance. And as everyone had predicted, I didn't give a damn who saw what.

"One more time, push, push, push!" the nurse shouted. At last, with a painful tear, the baby's head came out, the umbilical cord wrapped around his neck. The doctor told me to stop while she suctioned his airways and cut the cord. Then one last painful push and out came the shoulders and Scott was in the world: 7:06 p.m., June 22, 2006, two days before my forty-third birthday.

The doctor put him immediately on my chest. Scott cried softly as the nurse toweled him off, then he just started looking around, laid-back and interested from the beginning. "Hi, baby," I said in a soft, quavering voice. I wasn't aware of it, but photos show that I had tears running down my cheeks. He was alarmingly blue at first—"Is he the right color?" I asked—with fuzzy ears and big feet. In fact he was fuzzy other places, too. "He could use a back waxing," I joked a few minutes later, after he'd pinked up. I held him close, stroking his tiny head over and over.

I felt calm and content, wanting only to lie there with my new baby. But since I was on the regular labor and delivery floor they quickly starting pressuring me to get out of the room and make way for the next mom. Scott and I were bundled into a wheelchair to be taken to postpartum, but I couldn't sit up without passing out. The staff seemed puzzled and concerned. Abrupt change of plans: One nurse took Scott from me and another wheeled me on a gurney into the recovery room. I lay there barely able to maintain consciousness, feeling robbed of my baby and worried that he felt abandoned. I was also terrified that after all the joy and jolliness over the healthy baby, after my friends and the doctor and the doula had said their good-byes and gone home for supper, I would end up slipping quietly into death, unnoticed by the overworked recovery-room nurse.

It turns out I'd had some postpartum hemorrhaging and was faint and severely anemic from losing all that blood—not so uncommon—but they didn't tell me that until much later. Finally, at four in the morning, I was strong enough to be reunited with Scott, who apparently had slept the whole time. Once I got him back I did not let him go. I went to sleep with Scott snuggled on my chest. During meals he slept curled on my lap under the hospital tray with a paper napkin over his head. He pretty much never saw the inside of that hospital bassinet. After almost fifteen years of wanting him and two years of trying to conceive and waiting for this moment, I had my baby at last.

## HARD DELIVERIES AND POSTPARTUM CHALLENGES

My delivery was, by and large, incredibly easy, if you don't count the scary hemorrhaging incident, and I was lucky to have friends and family with me the entire time. But you never know what's going to happen, and as a single-mom-to-be, you won't necessarily have someone always at your side. That can be particularly hard during childbirth and the postpartum period. Most times, everything goes well, but it pays to be prepared for the possibility that it may not be smooth sailing.

The challenge may be a profound one. As with any birth, there's always the small chance the baby will have a major health or developmental problem. Ruth, a single mom by choice from Ohio, knows from experience that there are no guarantees. "I was the perfect pregnant person twice," she says, regarding the two kids she had by donor insemination. "No alcohol, no NutraSweet, no caffeine, I took all my vitamins, I exercised, etcetera. My oldest child is high-functioning autistic. My second has Crohn's disease and a number of learning differences." Ruth adopted a third child from an orphanage in Siberia. "My youngest, for whom we had very limited birth-parent information and who was institutionalized for the first two years of his life, has no issues," she says. Go figure. "Children are who they are, no matter how they arrive in your family," says Ruth, who, despite the challenges of raising special-needs kids, loves being a mom.

Coping with a seriously handicapped child as a single mom is beyond the scope of this book, though when you're considering single motherhood, it's important to realize it's a real possibility. But single moms can face more common challenges as well, like premature birth, labor complications, and twin births. According to a 2003 study published in the *American Journal of Public Health*, 43 percent of all women experience some type of health problem during their hospital stay—whether that means high blood pressure, a C-section, a bad tear, or hemorrhaging, like I had. The good news is that the percentage of women who have life-threatening complications is very low. I talked to a few women who had challenging experiences about what got them through—like reaching out for help and trying to keep a sense of humor.

When Cheri, nine months pregnant, went in for her final ultrasound, things looked really bad. "There was an erratic heartbeat, so they were going to induce." Though she received that frightening news alone, she had company soon enough. "God bless her, my friend came over as soon as she heard I checked into the hospital," Cheri says. Still, a labor-support friend isn't the same as a husband or partner. The induction wasn't going to start until the next morning, so the friend went home instead of staying over in the uncomfortable foldout guest bed. But in the middle of the night Cheri was told she needed to have an emergency C-section. She was all alone. "I ended up calling my friend at five in the morning, just bawling," Cheri says. "She came over, and my parents came over. It was really scary, being wheeled into the operating room, but my friend was with me. It was so cold my teeth were chattering." For Cheri, the C-section was surreal. "I remember my body moving as they pulled him out. It took me a long time to kind of process that experience." Cheri was terribly disappointed that she didn't get to have a vaginal birth, but the baby was healthy and the hospital staff was supportive. "The nurse said, 'You gave birth to this child. Don't you ever doubt it!' "

Amanda, who had been in the hospital for weeks with a rare pregnancy complication, had a scary birth, too. She had settled in to the hospital bed-rest routine, figuring she had at least a month to go, until one day a test showed the blood flow to the baby had become severely restricted and doctors abruptly told her, "Stop eating, we have to deliver the baby." That's when Amanda really got scared. She knew it was way too early for the baby to be born. The medical team delivered Amanda's daughter at twenty-six weeks (forty is normal). "She was actually crying when she was born, which doctors couldn't believe," Amanda says (lung function does not normally get to that point until much later). But at one pound, four ounces, little Leah was far from being out of the woods—she spent her first couple months in the neonatal intensive-care unit on a ventilator. And, as happens to many single moms, Amanda discovered some weak links in her support system.

"A twenty-six-week fetus does not look like a miniature version of a baby," Amanda says. "Her head was the size of the bottom of a Heineken bottle. The skin is all wrinkled and is this unnatural shade of pink. It's very hard to look at. A lot of people who were very good about coming to the hospital when I was there pregnant would take one look at the baby and say, 'I've gotta go.' My brother and some of my girlfriends ran for the hills." So Amanda was exhausted from the birth, worried sick about her daughter, and more alone than she would have anticipated.

That's where humor came in. Amanda has a dry, sarcastic wit, which kept her going through the challenges. For example, she just had to laugh about that fundamentalist Christian woman who thought baby Leah's problems were God's judgment on Amanda's choice. Wrath of God or not, she was definitely a wreck. "One day the doctor saw me in the hall and said, 'You don't use heroin, do you?' I said no. 'Well, you look like a heroin addict,' " joked the doctor. " 'Bathing hasn't been an option for you, has it? If you stand on a street corner with a cup, people will give you change.' "

Even once baby Leah got out of the hospital, the ordeal wasn't over. "She has so many special needs, my life does pretty much revolve around her," Amanda says. Leah receives physical therapy, occupational therapy, and speech/feeding therapy twice a week for a total of six sessions weekly. She's required two rounds of steroids and many rounds of antibiotic treatment. Her improperly developed nervous system means that she has some sensory issues, and "certain noises freak her out," Amanda says. Feeding has also been a challenge, since Leah got used to eating through a tube. Still, Amanda says, "she's a great little baby and I wouldn't trade her for the world. I love being a mom, I think it's the best thing." Luckily, Amanda says, Leah's special needs aren't that serious in the long run, though it may be eight years before Leah really catches up to children her age, according to the latest research on "micropreemies." "I think we'll be OK. She's got a couple of little problems, like minor damage to her peripheral vision, but nothing life-altering. And I have my own business, so I'm able to be flexible. I think we'll have a nice life together. Hopefully, in eight or ten years she'll be just another petite little girl. If not, well, we'll cross that bridge like we crossed many, many bridges so far!"

Though forty-six and pregnant with twins (something that happens fairly commonly to women who use fertility drugs or in vitro fertilization), Laura had a fairly uneventful, active pregnancy—she was able to take a challenging prenatal yoga class into her third trimester. But then, as with Amanda's experience having a preemie, things got bad. "The first few months were just insane," Laura says. "It's not for the faint of heart, being single with twins." One of the babies was breech, so Laura delivered by C-section. Her mom came to help her, but then when they were leaving the hospital her mom slipped and broke her hand. "She couldn't use her hands and I couldn't bend over and pick anything up." Then things got even crazier. "The second day after going home, my belly burst open," Laura says. When she went to the doctor, he opened the wound up all the way and said it had to stay open and be packed with fresh gauze on a regular basis. Oh, no, that wouldn't be me, Laura thought. I faint at the sight of blood. But there she was, in her own private horror movie—"My stomach was wide open," Laura says—and fainting was not an option. There was an upside to the gore. "My upstairs neighbor is a photographer and she's doing a project that involves wounds," Laura says, laughing about it now. "She thought it was horrible, so she came by with her camera to take pictures." It took the wound two months to heal, so in the meantime Laura was trying to lift the twins up over it to breast-feed. Her mom stayed for a few weeks and was able to be tremendously supportive emotionally, though physically, with her broken hand, "it was a disaster because everything she touched either fell or broke or spilled." She had to hire a baby nurse to help out.

All in all, says Laura, who is now wearing splints on both wrists because of the strain of handling the two babies, "it's been harder than I thought it would be. There's this whole maddening aspect when two babies are crying at once; you can't physically take care of them both at the same time. Pretty much, you can't sleep. There's always someone who needs to be fed. Even though I had a night nurse, I was breast-feeding so I was up all the time." Laura went for about three or four months without much sleep. "The level of pain is just beyond," she remembers. "It's just beyond. It's worse than anything I experienced in the hospital. There was a three- or four-day stretch when the nanny called in sick and I got three hours' sleep total." Without a partner, of course, there's no built-in emergency backup. "Every day it was like, 'What have I done? Will I live through it? Will my life ever be worth living again?'" Laura reached out, through the Single Mothers by Choice organization, to another single mother of twins, who assured her it would get better and, as for most parents of twins, it did. When I spoke to Laura, the twins were seven months old, she was back at work and getting six or seven hours of sleep a night. "I'm really starting to see the light at the end of the tunnel," Laura says. "I'm completely functional," she says, though until recently she has had help in the form of a night nurse twice a week. And Laura's starting to see having two as a benefit, since they can entertain each other. "Already if I leave the room, I face them to each other and they seem content."

## LIFE WITH A NEW BABY

Though the postpartum period can be hard, especially if you have multiples or a preemie, it can also be pretty easy. That's not something I expected—you always hear such horror stories about sleep deprivation and stress, right?—but that's how it was for me. It was that way for other single moms I've spoken to as well. So while you should always prepare for the worst, it's OK to also expect the best. Angela, who has two teenage kids, says new motherhood was not particularly hard for her. She remembers her postpartum period, spent mostly alone with son Robin, now seventeen: "Basically, I didn't really need any help, because he was breast-fed and so I didn't need anyone to help me sterilize bottles or anything." Angela was laid-back about it from the beginning, and didn't feel like she needed highly specialized skills or tools or information in order to take care of the baby. "I guess I kind of figured that people had been doing this a long time," she says. "We have lost touch with the joy and naturalness of it."

"Some of the books make it out to be harder than it is," says Suzie, in agreement. "Like you have to have people come over to help you bathe the baby. I've never had to have that. Just give 'em a bath!"

Kimberley took almost nine months off from work, and it was a wonderful, relaxing experience for her. "I loved Felix's babyhood," she says. "I was never miserable or lonely. I slept during the day, I watched soap operas, I never put myself down for anything."

I've always loved babies. Still, I fully expected that during those first weeks and months I'd feel overwhelmed and desperate at times, out of my mind with sleep deprivation or postpartum depression, caught on a hamster wheel of diaper changes and stabbed with loneliness every time the baby did something cute and I didn't have a partner to share it with. I felt sure I'd be like Anne Lamott, best-selling writer and single mom by accident, who wrote a month after her son was born, "I wonder if it is normal for a mother to adore her baby so desperately and at the same time to think about choking him or throwing him down the stairs." I mean, I certainly had moments of feeling murderous toward my beloved dog Ripley, especially when I came home after a stressful day to find the kitchen garbage strewn across the apartment. I figured a child wouldn't be all that different.

Instead, I became sort of a Stepford Mom, June Cleaver, Pollyanna parent. I don't know whether I was blissed out on breast-feeding hormones or finally getting what I'd spent almost fifteen years yearning for, but I was happy, happy, happy. I can't write this without rolling my eyes, but it's the truth: For the first couple months, at least, I felt honored to change Scott's diapers. Seriously. Even at four in the morning, after being up every two hours, I'd be confronted with a poopy diaper and I'd feel lucky. Having this beautiful little boy snuggled next to me in bed, looking up at me like I was the pot of gold at the end of the rainbow, I needed nothing else to make me happy. I had anticipated feeling sad that I didn't have someone to share the experience with, but I didn't feel that way at all. I felt like I'd welcomed a partner but I didn't feel like I needed one or lacked anything.

I would shed the occasional tear of joy and wonder, overwhelmed at how much I loved this little man. And I did cry sometimes, in sadness, because I suddenly knew how terribly short life is, that these moments would fly by, and I'd grow old and die and leave this precious boy forever. "Weeeeee may never pass this way again . . ." sang my hackneyed, maudlin, seventies-era subconscious as tears rolled down my cheeks.

Before I had Scott, I never understood why people talked in terms of "falling in love" with your baby. That's a romantic, sexual thing, I thought. Of course you *love* your child, but "in love"? I thought directing that phrase toward an infant was a little creepy, and definitely a little Hallmark—you know, characteristic of the kind of folks who send out those cards with sappy poetry printed in loopy script over soft-focus pictures of sunsets. Barf.

Now I understand. Loving your baby is almost exactly like the other kind of "in love." Here's this person I absolutely adore, who totally captivates me, who I look at and feel so happy and blessed to be spending time with, just the way I felt the last time I was in love. I may draw the line at soft-focus sunsets, but I'm on my way there. My subconscious, which has an embarrassing tendency to provide a really ham-handed sound track to my life, chose Simon & Garfunkel here: "Life I love you, all is groovy."

Though most moms seem to get to that nauseatingly "in love" place eventually, it doesn't always come so quickly. It's perfectly normal not to feel an immediate bond. Life with even a healthy infant can be a shock to the system, and falling in love can take time. "When Jack was first born, I was

amazed and in awe of him," says Cheri, "but I didn't feel that immediate connection. I spent the first few weeks just feeling like his concierge. It took a
while to feel like a mother."

Liz had that new-mom freakout a little when she was first alone with her
twin boys. "It's four in the morning after they clean up everything, then
they drop off these two alien creatures in the room, and they're like, bye!
And I'm like, you're kidding me! What am I supposed to do with them?!"

## UP YOUR ODDS OF AN EASY BABY

Scott was a naturally easygoing, happy baby, which I'd say was the number one reason why his infancy did not seem overwhelming to me. I
simply lucked out. Your baby's temperament is a huge factor in how hard
he is to deal with as a newborn, and there are many stories of smug parents
who had an easy first child, then got walloped with the second. But some
of the expert advice I heeded really made a difference, and there were some
reasons why suddenly having a baby to care for was not a shock to my
system. Though nothing will work for every baby or every mom, here's what
worked for me.

Easy Baby Rule Number One: *Don't freak out.* Like some other eldest-
daughter single moms I interviewed, I was very comfortable with infants. As
a result, I totally bypassed the New Parent Freakout Factor, which is, in my
opinion, the main reason first-time parents of healthy babies find parenthood
so hard. I have witnessed new parents as they struggle, and from what I have
seen it's often 20 percent perspiration, 80 percent hyperventilation. (You
rarely see anyone having such a hard time with baby number two.) If you're
seriously type A and need to hyperventilate to keep yourself entertained
during maternity leave, go right ahead. But my feeling is if you're going to
be a single mom, you don't have the luxury to freak out. You need to put that
energy elsewhere. So my best advice is read a good all-round infant-care
book (like Dr. William Sears's *Baby Book,* my fave, or *What to Expect the First
Year,* by Arlene Eisenberg, Heidi Murkoff, and Sandee Hathaway) and then
take a chill pill.

Rule Two: If you've never taken care of a newborn, for God's sake, practice! I had two little sisters for whom I was Mom Number Two, I babysat a
lot as a teenager, and more recently, I have taken care of my sister's three kids.

If you aren't so experienced, I'd urge you to find someone with an infant and beg for training in return for free babysitting.

Here's a cautionary tale: My upstairs neighbor's daughter-in-law came to visit Scott when he was a couple weeks old and she was about eight months pregnant with her first child. I asked if she'd like to hold the baby. She looked pale and nervous, but said sure. So I put Scott down and watched as she stood staring at him, apparently immobilized with fear, trying to figure out how exactly she was going to go about this tricky maneuver of picking up the infant. The conversation stopped. The baby lay there. She stood there, still staring at him, doing this little twitchy thing with her beautifully manicured hands and shifting from foot to foot. Finally Scott, feeling abandoned on his back and wanting to be held, had enough and started to cry. The soon-to-be mom recoiled as if she had seen a snake.

"Oh, he's not happy; I'll hold him another time," she said as she backed quickly out of the apartment. My mom and I laughed. To give the mom-to-be credit, she had just had her baby shower and may just have been emotionally wiped out, but I can only imagine the horror of being that inexperienced with babies and then being presented with one of your own!

Rule Three: If you're planning to breast-feed, learn about "latch-on"—that's the way in which the infant attaches to your nipple. Some friends of mine had nightmarish first weeks and months with their babies because of breast-feeding problems—terrible pain, cracked nipples, and mastitis infections, all of which lactation experts link to improper latch-on. I had always figured breast-feeding would go fine for me, but the horror stories scared me into taking a class. Now, every expert has a different theory on what's right and wrong, and the class I took was sort of like Breast-feeding for Drill Sergeants. Not exactly my style. I ended up discarding most of the advice, except for the one thing everyone agrees with: If you don't have a proper latch-on, you're screwed. And everyone seems to agree on the proper technique. So I made sure I knew exactly how Scott's mouth was supposed to fit over my nipple, and I didn't have any breast-feeding trouble or pain at all. Coincidence? Who knows—but I was glad I'd done what I could to increase my chances of having an easy time.

While breast milk is best for babies, it's important to note both that you can do everything right and still have problems and that not everyone is able to breast-feed. One friend of mine had one of those rare problems where she really didn't produce enough milk, despite trying for months with lots of professional help. It was heartbreaking for her, but it does happen to some women and their babies do just fine.

Rule Four: Think cozy. Babies like to be close to their moms. So let 'em, says one school of parenting. That theory made sense to me, and I think heeding it is part of why I had such an easy baby and such an easy transition into motherhood. I kept Scott close to me; he was happy and so was I. I also took some advice from my California ex-sister-in-law (who has two wonderfully well-adjusted kids) and slept with the baby next to me in bed, which meant that all I needed to do to breast-feed him all night was roll onto my side and stick a boob into his mouth. I'd be back asleep before he was finished, and I never felt sleep deprived. I talked to several other single moms who slept with their babies as infants—much easier when you're single and you don't have a spouse who might object to sharing the bed— and they also said they avoided sleep deprivation as a result. Enough sleep was and is my number one personal priority. The times I don't get enough sleep, suddenly parenting does seem bleak and overwhelming. In addition to sleeping with Scott, I also picked him up a lot, wore him in a sling carrier a lot (which was like baby Valium; many times he'd be inconsolable and the minute I put him in the sling he calmed right down), and fed him whenever he was hungry.

There's lots of debate about these practices, especially cosleeping—well-respected experts come down on both sides of the issue. For me the bottom line was that the ways of handling an infant I've just described have been the norm in most of the world for most of history. I have to assume it worked pretty well for all those mothers, and, boy, did it work well for me. Hopefully the approach will continue to bear benefits—there have been studies that show that babies that get what they want during early infancy are happier and less whiny and insecure as toddlers. I got criticism for my methods, mainly from my old-school mom, but I also constantly got compliments: "Wow, what an amazing baby. Does he *ever* cry?" More important, I had a happy, secure baby and we both got plenty of sleep.

Rule Five: See crying as a problem to solve. Scott wasn't always a suspiciously happy baby. But when he became colicky in his early weeks, instead of just accepting the dictum that "babies cry," I heeded one of my baby books and saw the crying as an indication that something was wrong. Infants don't *have* to be crybabies, the book suggested, so I did my best to find out what was hurting Scott, at one point cutting every possible irritant out of my diet.

According to the books I read, many young infants can't digest the protein in cow's milk, even when it comes to them through their mother's breast milk. In addition to milk, there was a long list of other foods that, when eaten by mom, could irritate a breast-fed baby. "So," I asked plaintively as I walked into a health-food store, "if you can't eat dairy or wheat or corn or oats or broccoli or beans, what's left?"

After some painful trial and error, I discovered Scott was definitely quite sensitive to cow's milk and probably also raw onion, raw garlic, and hot peppers. Bingo. Once I changed my diet, my baby pretty much stopped crying. And I had to wonder whether it was hereditary and whether, forty-three years earlier, my months of colic as a newborn were caused by the same simple—and apparently fairly common—cow's milk–protein sensitivity. Of course, as a milk and cheese addict, changing my diet was painful. I had to do it for eight months till he outgrew the problem—Scott's damn lucky I think he's cute.

Actually, we were both lucky I found the culprit. It's not always possible to figure out the reason the baby is hurting, so while it's good to try, it's not a good idea to make yourself crazy (see Elisa's story, on pages 225–27, for both what to do and what not to do).

Rules Six, Seven, Eight, Nine, and Ten: Don't get isolated. The other rules may just be my personal opinion (and that of my favorite experts), but pretty much everyone can agree on this one. Isolating yourself in your baby's first year is a great way to get depressed and go crazy. For a number of the single moms I spoke to, first-year isolation was one of the hardest things about single motherhood. This isn't specific to single moms by choice, though—from what I've seen, I'd say married moms are actually more likely to isolate themselves during maternity leave. They think they don't need to seek out as much socializing since they have their husbands. But after a few months of intense one-on-one with an infant, with a husband who comes home tired late at night, they end up feeling much more isolated than your typical single mom, who knows she needs to get out there. Still, not all single moms do take the initiative, and the result isn't pretty.

"During the four months that I was off on maternity leave I didn't have much adult contact," admits Debrah. "I probably would have someone over once a week. If I had to look back on it, I wouldn't recommend being with that child day and night and thinking of yourself as the only person who should be with him." At one point, Debrah's parents came to visit and administered a little tough love. "You *have* to schedule time away from him," they insisted. "They could see I was going nuts," she says.

There's an important distinction to be made between garden-variety "going nuts" and postpartum depression, which is a serious medical condition that should be treated immediately. If you find yourself feeling hopeless, depressed, or overwhelmed, be sure to alert your doctor as soon as possible.

Julie, who's a very social person, knew she had to stay connected. "I made sure I had plans to do something or see someone every day, or I knew I'd be depressed," she says. It wasn't always easy, though—Julie had a bulky stroller that wasn't exactly designed to take into the New York City subway system. "My legs were so bruised all summer," Julie remembers, laughing. "I was pretty strong, I guess." She'd go to friends' houses, or out to dinner, and the baby would just sleep in the stroller or on a friend's bed. "Milo was an easy child, easy to pick up, package up, and take along." Even so, Julie says, she felt quite lonely in that postpartum period. "I didn't want to bore my friends with cute little things he did," she says, and she was surprised at how much she missed having someone to share those things with.

Robin, mom of five-year-old Fred, counsels single moms to get out there. "You tend to want to isolate yourself, because you have to feed the kid every two hours, but go out to the park, introduce yourself," Robin says. Before your baby comes, find out—by asking moms or asking at baby boutiques—what your options will be. Perhaps there's a coffee shop or playground or bookstore where new moms tend to hang out. For me it was incredibly easy because I moved into a neighborhood so family-friendly that childless people snipe about "stroller gridlock," where a local maternity store organizes New Mom groups, and where one of the coffeehouses often looks more like a playground. But if there isn't anything like that in your area, you can start a mom's group by posting flyers in places pregnant women might be.

Kimberley took full advantage of her son Felix's portability when he was an infant. "I took him everywhere with me. He lived in a Baby Björn for the first six months of his life," she says. "Every picture of him is me with a napkin over his head, eating. I went out to dinner all the time at people's houses and I visited friends out of state. He slept in the bed with me so I didn't have to bring much. At about five months I put him into the crib." For her, being single during that period was a big plus. "You get to just sleep whenever you want and there's no 'What about our marriage?'"

One big factor in avoiding isolation as a new single mom is location, location, location. That may be something to consider carefully before embarking on the single-motherhood journey. When her daughter was first born, Jocelyn lived in a town house. "It was really not a child-oriented community, to say the least," she says. "When my daughter was really young I got stir-crazy. I used to go to McDonald's playland and read books just to be around other people." Finally, she decided she needed to make a change. "I picked a school district and I drove around looking for a neighborhood that had a lot of kids. On this one street I had to go about three miles an hour because there were so many kids, so I bought a house on that street."

The change really paid off. "I met other mothers, and I'd tell parents, if you ever want to go out, leave your kids with me. And I figured in a pinch, they'd do the same for me—and they did."

## CREATIVE WAYS TO AVOID ISOLATION

My friends in lesbian couples were by and large quite traditional and regimented with their infants, suddenly spending all their nights at home, their babies bathed and put to bed with Swiss-watch punctuality. One good friend told me, as if this was just part and parcel of being a parent, that she and her partner really didn't see most of their nonparent friends anymore—their new life was all about the baby and hanging out with other parents. That's cool, I guess, if it's what you want and if you have a partner to keep you company. But being a single mom by choice is unconventional. For me, it's also made sense to dispense with other baby-related conventions that don't work, especially when there doesn't seem to be a real reason to comply. This has been a lifesaver for me in the first year. I haven't really felt bored, isolated, or depressed at all, and the closing down of social options that comes with motherhood has happened in a more gradual, comfortable way. For example, infants are supposed to be up at dawn and in bed by seven o'clock, right? Well, I haven't had that kind of schedule since high school—standard business hours for magazine editors are ten to six—and I wasn't eager to start, unless there was a real reason for it, like school hours or Scott himself requiring it. At least for the first nine months, Scott was happy to join me in my freelancer's schedule of staying up late and sleeping late. (It took a little encouragement—at six weeks he started to think five o'clock in the morning was kick and play time, but I was able to convince him otherwise by pretending I was asleep. Soon he gave up and happily joined me in slumber.)

Another convention is that babies are supposed to lie around in their pastel nurseries, stimulated only by plastic objects that have been produced by Fisher-Price or entertained with electronic singing by Elmo. But keeping baby tucked away in a nursery is just another middle-class Western tradition, one that may not work well for anyone—babies are isolated and bored, stay-at-home moms go stark raving mad, and everyone else lives an utterly child-free existence until such time as they switch to an insanely child-centered one. Women have gone about their business with babies strapped to them for thousands of years. So, especially in the first six months, I took Scott with me everywhere, unless it was a formal party or it would otherwise be disruptive or inappropriate. If in doubt, I'd ask if it was OK, and usually it was. It was never disruptive—if Scott started to cry, I'd leave immediately. As a babe in arms, Scott wasn't underfoot (crawlers and toddlers are a lot less easy to bring along), and he was either fascinated by the lights and the people, or he would fall asleep in his sling, happy to be with Mom. At parties, people either seemed delighted to see the baby or they just ignored him. Sometimes they wouldn't even realize I had a baby with me, mistaking his sling for a large purse. Occasionally I'd get the kind of look you might get if you were attending an event with your six-foot-long pet boa constrictor around your neck, but that was rare. Scott loved parties unless they were too loud, generally enjoyed going out for restaurant dinners, and loved going to visit friends in their apartments. And some people, like the members of my writer's group, were amazing about accommodating Scott (plus, I think they kind of liked having a baby around). As a result, I was able to continue to meet with them without having to fork over fifty dollars for a babysitter.

By not making assumptions about what life with a newborn "should" be, I was able to create a life that was fun for both of us. My friends helped. A few days after I returned to Brooklyn from the summer in Maine, Scott and I went out to dinner in the East Village with my friend Sally, and then we went back to her house for a movie. Sally and I talked late into the night, and by the time I was ready to leave it was two in the morning—not a great time to use the subway. Sally told me I should stay over on her sofa bed.

An impromptu sleepover? With a two-month-old infant? I'd never heard of such a thing. But when I thought about it, me, my breasts, and enough diapers and wipes (I had to buy more at the drugstore the next morning) were all Scott really needed. We had a great sleep on Sally's pullout couch with her dog Dotty curled protectively at our feet, and then we all went out to brunch the next morning. Scott had a grand old time, and seemed thrilled to get out of the suburbs.

Three weeks after Scott was born, at the invitation of my friend Kevin, I had boarded the subway and taken the baby to my regular Tuesday night swing dance to introduce him to all the people who had seen him grow in my belly for nine months. Kevin held him while I danced a couple dances, though I was still very weak and sore, so I didn't do much. I then went to stay with my mom for a couple months, but when I got back I went to the dance again, with Kevin as my "dance nanny," figuring it was just this once. It worked really well, though, and Scott seemed to love the music and the movement. So I asked the dance studio owner if I could come regularly, so long as Scott was not fussy or crying. "Sure!" she said. "We'd love him to come!" I'd have to hustle him out of there if he started to fuss, she said, but otherwise it was fine. More than fine. "You can take classes if you want," she said.

Dance class? With an infant in tow? Was she insane? I was sure that wouldn't work, but what the hell, I had to try it. I double-checked with the teacher, who was delighted to have the baby attend, and gave it a shot, parking Scott in his stroller with some toys while I took class. Scott loved it! Sometimes even if he'd had a bad day, dance class would perk him right up. He seemed fascinated with the dancing and the music, and when there were too many women in the class he'd hold court, flirting with them while they waited their turn for a partner. Sometimes I'd have to stop and nurse him, but not that often. Not once did I have to leave because of a squalling baby. It worked for months, until Scott started crawling, and gave both of us a lot of pleasure.

I started to refer to the lindy-hop class as "Scott's office hours." After class, we'd go to the practice dance, and Kevin and I (and often others) would take turns holding him and dancing. This meant that every Tuesday night of his infancy Scott got to go out swing dancing, being bounced to the likes of Louis Armstrong and Lionel Hampton instead of lolling around listening to Barney and Elmo. Scott adored the activity and attention, and by six and a half months a few people swore he'd started to kick his feet to the beat. And something else happened—many of the dancers got used to Scott being there and really missed him when we didn't show up.

New York City probably provides many more opportunities for including an infant in a parent's activities than most suburban areas do, and my flexible schedule obviously gave me a lot of freedom, too. If I'd had to be at work at nine, dancing till ten-thirty the night before would not have been possible. But I'd urge other single moms to keep an open mind about what the requirements of infant care really are and to take advantage of opportunities to do things other than stay at home and bond with Barney. Of course, even though most infants are highly portable, you can't do everything you used to do, both for the sake of those around you and for the sake of the child. Also, different babies can have very different needs. I make sure that whatever the activity is, it's working for Scott and he's not unhappy or overwhelmed. Psychotherapist and single mom Jane Mattes, author of *Single Mothers by Choice*, says that's key—single moms trying to maintain a social life sometimes can be tempted to think of their kids as "little adults" and include them in activities that are not developmentally appropriate for them. Examples of that would be taking a three-year-old to an R-rated film (I see coupled parents do this, too!) or taking a toddler to a full-length ballet and expecting him to behave well.

I take my cue from my baby. If something works for both of us, great. If it works for me but not for him, he wins. When Scott was about three months old, my friends with an older baby invited me to Baby Loves Disco, a kids' party held in a beer-soaked bar in my neighborhood. But the music was overwhelmingly loud and Scott wasn't happy, so even though I wanted to hang out with my friends I took him straight out of there. But Scott and I are not the only factor in these equations. If something works for Scott and me but not for the people around us, they win. I try to be aware of whether or not we might be bothering anyone, and if there is the slightest chance we are, I leave. Now that Scott's crawling and walking, there are a lot of things I don't take him to that I would have when he'd just lie in his sling and look cute. But if Scott's welcome, will have fun, and won't be a burden, I bring him!

## WHAT A SUPPORT SYSTEM IS—AND ISN'T

Do you have a good support system?" everyone asks when they find out you're planning single motherhood.

"What the hell does that mean?" I've always wanted to know. People say it as if they're asking some perfectly straightforward question, like whether or not you have good health insurance. "Why, yes," I imagine the perfect answer goes, "I finalized the two-year contracts last week. Suzie has agreed to drop everything and start making chicken soup anytime I have the sniffles, Bob has signed up for any heavy lifting or childproofing that needs to be done, Amy is cheerfully standing by for hysterical phone calls in the middle of the night, Evan will babysit whenever I need, I've scheduled Tim to come by three times a week to give me a neck rub, and Mimi has bought a pager so she can rescue me if I find myself in town with too many shopping bags." Maybe some people have this kind of community, but I don't. Also, even if you are so lucky, can you really know it beforehand and count on it as part of your official plan? I don't think so. Besides, not even partnered moms-to-be can necessarily count on anything. Partners and husbands take off, die—like my dad did when my mom was six months pregnant with my brother—or, more commonly, just fail to be of much help.

Charlene, the educational consultant with the four-year-old daughter, found her support system wasn't quite what she'd hoped. She thought she knew what single motherhood was going to mean, but she was still surprised. When she had her baby, her mom, who hadn't slept in three days, had a ministroke and was unable to help. And her best friend was a busy small-business owner who couldn't deal with Charlene's choosing single motherhood because it made her reflect on her own single, childless status. "Here I was sick, I had had a C-section, they had to put me under and I almost bled to death. At one point, my doctor realized that I was alone. That sort of stunned her. She said, 'But you could die." I really needed help. It was then that I realized what it was like to be by myself, one thousand percent."

Charlene needed to stay in bed for six weeks, and she did come up with some work-arounds. She hired a doula. Another friend finally came through for her, even though she had a partner at home. And a community of acquaintances pitched in. "I knew the people at the pizzeria and the chicken place and they made special less-seasoned food for me," Charlene says.

After her experience, Charlene recommends having fewer expectations but keeping an open mind and a hopeful attitude. "Be open to the possibilities," she says, "because people are great. My neighbors came through for me. People I worked with came through for me. But my friends did not. I did not expect that. When the baby became real, it became a problem." To make matters worse, Charlene suffered from postpartum depression. "Now, I wouldn't give my daughter up for the world. But to be that alone, because your friends are dealing with their own issues, that was scary. It was so not what I expected, to be that alone."

Some of that aloneness is just the way it is to be a single mother. Even if they don't come through on a regular basis, most spouses will come through in a real pinch, Charlene points out. But "when you're by yourself, your child is with you. If you have to go to the hospital with asthma at one in the morning, who do you call? Yeah, you can call a friend, but you're less likely to," she says. As well meaning as they might be, other people have their own lives and their own problems to attend to, and as a single mom, you're the only one absolutely dedicated to your child. When this reality first hit Charlene, it was a shock.

Rachel is another single mom by choice who thought she'd have more support than she ended up having. "A lot of my friends and people I thought would be supportive sort of fell away," she says. In retrospect, she suggests doing more homework before the baby comes, "checking out child-care situations, really talking to your good friends about how involved they can be, and learning to ask for help."

Back in 1996, I'd had a snowboarding accident that taught me a hard lesson about single life and support systems. It took almost two years for me to recover from the head injury, and for the first few months I was, as I jokingly put it at the time, "somewhat vegetative." I assumed my close friends would rally, check in on me, bring me soup, whatever. Didn't happen. A few folks I thought were my closest friends turned out to be more accurately in the "fun people to see a movie with" category. The casual friends I saw movies with were, well, at the movies. With healthy people. I got the most support from my ex Joan (I call her Glinda the Good Ex), even though she had dumped me six months earlier. Then I got support from the most unlikely places, like this guy I had dated briefly a few months before the accident. David barely knew me and the romantic moment was over for both of us. Still, he'd call me every week or so to see how I was. It was sweet and unexpected. But more to the point, it was more than many of my supposedly good friends were doing. Mostly, though, I tried to get by without help, which in retrospect was insane and risky. Not only did I put myself through needless physical and emotional exhaustion, but I could have been killed—I was dizzy and out of it, and there were times where it really wasn't safe for me to cross a busy street by myself.

I learned a couple things from that experience. One, you really gotta ask for help. (Do I? Not often, but I am getting better at it, I swear.) And two, you really can't know in advance who's going to be there for you. If you make assumptions, you may be terribly disappointed, which leaves you both on your own *and* emotionally devastated. So, going into the single motherhood experience, my answer to the "support system" question was, "I don't know. We'll see!"

It has worked out exactly like that. Once again, a few of the people I might have assumed would be there for me in a bigger way were almost entirely missing in action. And once again, help and support has come from the most unexpected of places.

Like June Gorman. In the 1978–79 school year, when I was in tenth grade, June was a senior and captain of the basketball team. I didn't think June even knew I was alive at the time, and she hadn't seen me in twenty-seven years. But when she heard I was having a baby as a single mom, she sent me a beautiful handmade baby blanket.

Then there's my friend Kevin, originally just an acquaintance from dance class. He barely knew me, but he was the only person besides my mother who made a point of calling to check in a couple times a week during my pregnancy: "Hi, honey. How you doing?" Then when Scott was born, he and his partner, Jeff, were literally the only friends who offered to babysit. Which they did, taking care of Scott at the dance studio every Tuesday night while I danced. Almost every week they'd have me over for dinner afterward, too, knowing that I was probably starved for adult company (I was). They'd make a bed of towels on the floor of their tiny Manhattan apartment, and when the baby would fuss Jeff would make his Coyote hand puppet sing "Somewhere Over the Rainbow" and Scott would stare at the puppet, entranced.

Of course, there were many times that old friends really came through. I had an amazing tree the Christmas I was pregnant because Amanda and Melissa drove me to the tree lot, carried the ten-foot balsam up three flights of stairs and struggled with the tree stand while I stood and watched. Sally went with me for my amniocentesis, marveled as Scott kicked and waved on the sonogram during the amnio, then tucked me into bed and fed me supper afterward. (It was also Sally who gave Scott his in-utero nickname, Fluffy, because she thought he looked like a kitten on an early sonogram.)

A week before the baby came, my friend Amy left her partner and two-year-old son in Rhode Island to come down and help me. She organized my nursery better than I ever could have, made lasagna for the freezer, and even cooked and hosted a dinner party for me. My friend Rose called me period-ically during my pregnancy and gave me so many hand-me-downs from her daughter Luna that, between her and my sister Isabel, who has three kids, I barely needed to buy anything. And when I asked my friend and former boss Anne and her husband, David, for a ride home from the hospital for Scott and me, they not only drove me home and helped me up the stairs, but Anne also put me to bed, unpacked my bags, did two loads of laundry, and fixed me a dinner tray. It was just exactly what I needed.

In fact, every single one of my friends was supportive of my pregnancy—I had none of the jealousy or judgment that some other single moms by choice have complained of. In the scheme of things, I was one of the lucky ones. Still, my policy of not expecting any help has served me well. A friend might do something amazing and generous, then not be heard from for four months. And that's OK. I chose to have a baby alone, and my friends, how-ever well meaning, have their own lives and concerns. I don't resent it when help and support and companionship don't come—and the reality is that they often don't—and I am so very grateful when they do.

There are definitely times that I should ask for help and I don't, out of stubbornness and pride, and sometimes the results are disastrous, like that ter-rible time during my pregnancy when I was in the hospital alone. Other times, going it alone feels good. Like the brand-new crib that arrived when Scott was two months old. It was really a two-person job, but I didn't feel comfortable asking anyone to help. So, with Scott either beside me or sleep-ing at the other end of the baby monitor, I hauled the big pieces up three flights of stairs, figured out a way to do the assembly job alone, put it together, and then broke down the five thick boxes it came in, sliced and folded them till they were regulation size, bundled them for recycling, and took them out to the garbage area. Once I was finished I was exhausted but feeling pleased with myself, like I was Rosie the Riveter.

Some single moms really don't have to go it alone, because they have a coparenting donor, or daily family support, or incredibly dedicated friends. Alice is one of the lucky ones. "I have more support than most married mothers," she says. "My mother is my partner in raising this baby." Her mom and her dad, who is very ill and needs care, moved in with her, and her brother has moved in as well to care for her dad. Alice and her mom are primary caretakers for her son, but Alice's brother is also around on a daily basis. "I am *not* by myself," Alice is careful to say. She is a single mom only in that she does not have a husband. "The women who are really going it alone? That's not for me," she says. "I could not raise a child by myself. If my mother died, I'd do what I needed to do, but I would not have chosen to raise a child alone."

Lisa M. also has a strong network of support. Her large and close-knit family all live nearby. "If I want to go out to the movies," she says, "I can call my phone tree and say, 'I need some Lisa time,' and they'll say, 'Sure, bring the kids over.' "

And Diana had the kind of support system everyone dreams of. That was at least in part due to how active she'd been in her community. "I'd been very involved in the community, working with children and families, teaching Hebrew school every Tuesday afternoon." So when she had her first baby, there was a community response. "I wrote one hundred forty thank-you notes, if that tells you anything," she says. "I never ate at home for two months after the baby was born," she says. "People would ask if they could bring food, and I'd ask, 'Can I come over to your house?' People volunteered to babysit, helped me learn how to soothe the baby." Perhaps Diana could hear the envy in my silence on the other end of the phone, because she quickly added, "Since then my circle has been a little smaller." OK, then.

## THE RISKS OF *NOT* ASKING FOR HELP

It's debatable whether I should have indulged myself in my Rosie the Riveter crib-assembling moment. I could have hurt myself or damaged the crib; anyone could see it was a two-person job. And I'm certainly not alone—many of the single moms I spoke to say they feel uncomfortable asking for help. It figures, I guess. If we were dependent, helpless types we probably wouldn't have dared to become single mothers in the first place. But Elisa was truly Rosie Run Amok. I hope her story shows how important it can be for a single mom to seek help when she really needs it, especially with a new baby.

"I knew having a baby would be harder than I could ever imagine," Elisa says, "but I went into it believing if there's a will, there's a way." Elisa has since decided there's a point at which all the will in the world doesn't cut it, and that there are some things you really can't handle just by powering through on your own. After a happy, easy pregnancy, Elisa entered a postpartum nightmare with her daughter Skye. "It was a real wake-up call," Elisa says, referring to her former belief that she could handle anything. "Without exaggerating, Skye would scream sixteen to eighteen hours a day, and she would only sleep for an hour or two at a time. If she was awake, she was crying." Elisa did not want to just let the baby scream all by herself; she felt the crying meant that something was wrong, and that she should be there to comfort her daughter. But when, day after day, the baby screamed and Elisa got no sleep, she did not call anyone for help. She did think something was seriously wrong with the baby, though, and went again and again to the pediatrician, only to be shrugged off as "an overwhelmed single mother, just complaining," and told "it's colic." Elisa knew better. "She wasn't OK and no one was listening." After the little girl endured seven weeks of agony, another doctor found the problem. "There was a webbing between her colon and her rectum that didn't dissolve," Elisa says. "She physically couldn't poop. She could have died." Skye had had only sporadic and very liquid bowel movements, which Elisa had been told was OK. It most certainly wasn't. The diagnosing doctor was furious that it hadn't been caught earlier.

Still, after the procedure, the baby kept crying. Elisa doesn't know why; perhaps she was just a high-needs infant to begin with, or perhaps the colon problem dragging on so long made her more sensitive and prone to cry. Whatever it was, Elisa didn't get a break and was up most of the time, 24/7 holding and rocking the crying baby. Meanwhile, she was having terrible breastfeeding problems. "I was constantly black and blue and had an infection," she remembers. Still, Elisa did not get help. "I was too pigheaded. I thought it was too expensive to hire help and I thought I could handle it," Elisa says.

Turns out, she couldn't handle it. "I thought the emotional aspect would be the hardest," she says. "But it was the physical. My body completely broke down." Elisa ended up in the hospital: "I blew four disks in my back." And, without any coherent support system set up in advance, she had to leave her daughter with a young babysitter who confided, as Elisa was on her way to have surgery, that she was bipolar and had stopped taking her medication. Fortunately, her daughter survived that sitter.

Finally, after months of toughing it out, Elisa asked for help—she posted on the Single Mothers by Choice Listserv that she was "losing it." It was her salvation. "Moms that I did not know came in and helped me, held the baby for me," she says. "This mom I didn't know came and brought me a dozen roses and a pound of Starbucks coffee, cleaned my bathroom, and left." Others would come by for three or four hours on a Saturday and hold the baby while Elisa showered or slept. And eventually, her daughter grew out of the problem. "She's amazing," Elisa says now. "She's definitely an independent, high-spirited kid, but she's so joyful." The joy now makes up for the pain, but "the part where I thought I might die lasted eight months," Elisa recalls.

"I think you can step up to the challenge," she says, "but motherhood is not for everybody. I know some moms with husbands and help whose babies just have colic and they can't handle it." Elisa's advice now? "As much as you think you don't have money for help, have someone in place beforehand and have them come help you. Find the money to get help. Or, if you don't want to leave your baby with anyone, at least pay for someone to come and cook food and clean your bathroom." And realize a half-crazed, exhausted-to-the-point-of-breakdown mother doesn't do your baby any good. Elisa now understands that her inability to ask for help really put herself and her baby at risk. Part of the reason she didn't was because she felt, as a single mother by choice, that "I did this to myself," therefore she did not have the right to ask for help. "I thought that when you're in a couple, you almost have more of a right to ask for help. Anyone can see that's wrong, but the idea is hard to unlearn."

Another reason Elisa didn't get help was because she was overwhelmed and she hadn't set up anything in advance. "If you don't have family around you, you should really look into what your community has to offer *before* you have the baby," says Robin, mom of five-year-old Fred, who is active in the Single Mothers by Choice support community and has extended a helping hand to overwhelmed new moms. "It can be hard to find resources when you're in a postpartum depression with a colicky kid and sure could use a break." It's best to line up help in advance for the first couple weeks, when you might be very weak from delivery or have terrible trouble nursing, but it's essential to at least figure out who you can call for help should you need it. You can't always depend on friends and family, as some single moms have discovered, but you can line them up the best you can, get involved with a support group before you actually need support, and find out in advance what your options might be. In addition to getting help from friends and family, you can hire baby nurses and postpartum doulas to help you with the baby, and lactation consultants to help you with any nursing issues. La Leche League, the nursing activist organization, will advise you for free. And it may be a good idea to see, in advance of any problems, if your community offers respite child care for emergency situations.

## THE DIFFERENCE HAVING CHILD CARE CAN MAKE

Having the financial ability to get help can really make a huge difference in the experience of single motherhood. For Mikki, who lost her twelve-hour-a-day job when she went on maternity leave, life with baby was much easier than the life she'd led before. "My first year after my daughter was born, I just felt more rested than I had for years." But the money Mikki had saved from having had such a high-powered job was a big reason for the restfulness. Not only was she financially able to stay home, but she had hired a three-day-a-week nanny who cooked and cleaned.

As Mikki discovered, a support system can be bought, to some degree. "I don't have too much of a support system," says Marcy, who lives in a navy town three thousand miles away from her friends and family, "but I have a great, great day-care provider." I do, too. My mom helped me with shopping and cooking the first two months of Scott's life, but I had no help at all the last seven weeks of my maternity leave. It went fine, but by the time I hired a part-time nanny when Scott was three and a half months old so I could get back to work, I was definitely happy for the break. It's hard to be a great parent if you're literally never away from your child. At the same time, as any mom can tell you, leaving your baby with a nanny or at day care for the first time can be like losing a limb.

"One of the hardest things was having to leave my child with a nanny," says Suzie. But having a nanny has made single motherhood a lot easier for her. "My nanny's like a wife. She does the shopping, cooking, and cleaning, and lets me feel like I can have quality time with the kids when I get home."

While some moms feel leaving a kid with a sitter is always second best, other moms feel the opposite—that having other caregivers actually enriches a child's life. "The more good people in a child's life, the better," says Debrah, mom to a three-year-old. She says she's never been afraid that child care is a bad thing for her son. And for Debrah, the balance is a good one. "When I finished maternity leave at four months, I couldn't wait to get back to work. But at the end of the day, I can't wait to get home and see him."

Some single moms with nannies end up developing more of a partnership with their caregiver than they might have otherwise. Debrah says she has a closer relationship with her nanny than she probably would if she were married. "When I do things, I include the nanny quite intimately in the decisions. For example, when I went to interview the preschool, I included the nanny." For a single mom, the nanny's the only other person who knows how your child is doing on an intimate, daily basis, and (presumably) cares. That's potent stuff—or at least for me it is. My part-time nanny and I exchange details of my son's day, the things he's learned, any health concerns, both of us speaking of him with love and pride and concern. I have read of married working moms feeling threatened by their kids' attachment to the nanny, but for me, it's all positive. I think it's good for him to have another caring adult around who's different from me, and it's definitely good for me to have another adult to talk to who cares for him. Though it's ultimately a professional relationship, not a personal one, I'm sure I would feel much more isolated if I did not have her as a partner in child rearing.

## OTHER CHALLENGES: "HELP" FROM FRIENDS, FAMILY, AND STRANGERS

Oh my God, the unsolicited advice you get as a new parent! Much of it is well meaning, I guess. But people butt in and criticize parenting in a way you just don't see happening on any other topic. I've had strangers say to me, an authoritative edge to their voice, "You're breast-feeding, of course?" and also (different strangers), on witnessing me breast-feeding, equally concerned and authoritative, "You feed him a bottle, too, right?" Now, that's *perfect strangers*—let's not even talk about what friends feel comfortable saying. "You better start doing X!" Or, "If you don't stop doing Y, you'll be sorry!"

All moms have to endure this kind of unwanted advice and criticism, particularly in the first year. But I do think it's worse for single moms. In the ideal partnership, a married or partnered mom has someone to back her up, or at least to bitch to about all the attacks—oops, I mean advice—she's being subjected to. If you're single, you're a sitting duck.

"People assume you need more advice because you're alone," agrees Amanda. For her, it was particularly irritating because of her premature, special-needs baby. Her daughter's needs and development were quite different from other babies', and so it wasn't just difference of opinion—the advice givers quite literally did not know what they were talking about. Still, they were full of advice and judgment, telling Amanda she was being overprotective or that her baby, who was developmentally delayed, wasn't rolling over because she was "lazy."

"I feel that people give advice *much* more freely to single women," says Kimberley. And she feels that the unwanted advice is harder to brush off—you don't have a husband or partner telling you to just ignore the idiots and joining you in a united front: "As a single person, you don't get to say 'We've decided,' " Kimberley says. "When you have a husband or partner, you can have steady ground with him."

The most interesting book of the many I've read on the subject of all the high-disagreement baby issues—sleeping, eating, crying—is *Our Babies, Ourselves* by Meredith Small, recommended to me by another single mom by choice (thanks, Janet!). This fascinating book, a window into the field of ethnopediatrics written for a popular audience, looks not only at warring U.S. baby research and experts but also at infant-rearing practices cross-culturally and through a variety of lenses—anthropology, sociology, medicine, and evolutionary biology. The bottom line is, whatever you do, you can't win—someone's always going to criticize your parenting choices. One of my favorite anecdotes from that book is about a U.S. anthropologist and her infant daughter who visit an obscure tribe of hunter-gatherers living in the forests of Paraguay, a culture in which, traditionally, *they don't tell people what to do.* Yet the minute she gets there she's taken aside by horrified and concerned tribeswomen for a lecture on all the things she's doing wrong as a mother!

Friends, strangers, and Paraguayan tribeswomen are the least of most single mom's worries, though, since unsolicited advice is often most freely given by family members. For me, that was the biggest postpartum challenge I faced. Now, I would never have given up those first eight weeks with Scott and my mom. I loved seeing her talk to him, and I have this adorable picture of one-week-old Scott talking back to her, his expression intent, his mouth looking like he's really telling her a thing or two. The three of us had some great times together. Mom taught me all the words to "Tea for Two" and accompanied me on the piano as I sang and made Scott's little legs dance the old soft shoe. When he was fussy Mom would play the piano and I'd hold Scott in my arms, swinging and bouncing him to the beat as I danced a vigorous version of the Alley Cat, an old line dance from 1962, the tempo getting faster and faster until I couldn't keep up anymore and Scott was happy again. I have a picture of baby Scott nestled in the crook of Mom's left arm, watching her, fascinated, as the fingers of her right hand move over the black and white keys.

It was wonderful to have the company, someone to have meals with, someone who cared about the baby and was actually interested in the state of his bottom and the color of his poop. It was nice having someone to laugh with me at the fact that the minute I wanted to eat, preferably just as I was sitting down to a major knife-and-fork dinner, Scott wanted to eat, so I'd have to nurse him and look longingly at the steak as it got cold. It never failed. And it was great to have help, particularly since I was quite weak from losing so much blood in delivery. For the first month, my mom did all the shopping and most of the cooking.

But there was a flip side.

"He's not even allowed to squeak and you pick him up. He'll never learn how to soothe himself! You're going to be sorry. Babies cry, Louise. They need to exercise their lungs. You're feeding him *again?!* I had four children and they all ate every four hours. You need to put him on a schedule. You're not going to give him a bath every day? When was the last time you bathed him?"

Yes, like many, if not most, grandmothers, my mom felt I was doing things wrong—chiefly that I held the baby too much and didn't allow him to cry. This was bound to create a spoiled, whiny, demanding monster incapable of soothing or amusing himself. I was on a path to ruining my life and his character, and she was seriously concerned. I explained that I understood her concerns but that I had different ideas, ideas that were backed up not only by my instinct but also by recent scientific and medical research. Nevertheless, she continued to be appalled, and according to one of my sisters, so was the rest of the family. Newborns are supposed to start developing independence and detaching from their mothers ASAP, they felt, and babies are supposed to and in fact *need* to cry, both to exercise their lungs and to get a jump on learning to stop being such, well, *babies*. (Did I mention that we're WASPs?)

After about six weeks of being kindly but constantly criticized, either aloud or silently, on this and a few other issues (for example, I fed Scott when he was hungry, which was every two hours, another no-no), I became quite depressed and overwhelmed. I still thought I was doing things right. I was getting nothing but compliments from friends and strangers: "Wow, you're so at ease with the baby, it's like you already have kids, you look great, you're dressed and out of the house, you're at the beach, you're so brave/energetic/relaxed, all I could do was lie on the couch for the first couple months. . . ." I felt things were going fantastically, I was thrilled to be a mom, I wasn't feeling particularly sleep deprived, everything felt easy and natural and good. But my mother was the closest thing to a partner I had, the person whose opinion meant the most to me. And she thought I was making terribly wrong parenting choices and seemed concerned about my mental and physical health because I didn't have the energy or desire, a month postpartum, to have more than a couple of major out-of-the-house activities each day, since I was awake every two hours at night to feed the baby and still suffering from mild anemia.

It's really standard grandmotherly behavior. I know another new mom, a married one, who told me she was relieved when her mom left, because the criticism was getting to her—and she listed the exact same litany of perceived transgressions (picking up the baby too much, feeding baby too often, sleeping with baby) that my mom had been after me about. It's their way of showing they care. But when you have a husband or partner, either your mom is not with you for as long or she's staying nearby, and in any case you've got your other half to back you up or to bitch to. Since I didn't have backup, the criticism that might have just become a good mother-in-law joke between me and my spouse turned out to be by far the hardest thing I have had to deal with as a single mom. I called a few friends and my ex-sister-in-law, whose parenting choices were even further away from my mom's than mine were, and talking to them helped me get over the frustration. Still, when I was finally home in Brooklyn and alone with Scott, I didn't feel overwhelmed to suddenly be without help—I felt relaxed and relieved. I could feed and hold my baby whenever I wanted without fear of judgment.

Kimberley, mom of a fourteen-month-old, points out that many single moms end up sharing much more of their parenting experience with their own mothers than they would if they were part of a couple. But grandmothers are grandmothers—they're from a different generation and so they're not always going to give you the kind of support your same-generation partner would. "We open ourselves up to sharing things and then we get shot in the foot," Kimberley says. She cited one experience she had with her own mom. She'd decided against circumcising her son. Kimberley's mother disagreed with the idea, and could not shut up about it. "It consumed her, constantly!" Kimberley says. "Finally I said, 'Why do you always want to talk about my baby's penis?' " Kimberley's mom snapped, "That's not funny!" but backed off a little after that.

The upshot is that, though some help is crucial for most new moms, having a new baby may not be as hard as you think it's going to be, and having family help may be harder than you anticipate. Coming up with a flexible plan may be a good idea, if that's possible. And it pays to be realistic about what it may be like to have another adult with her own routines and opinions suddenly sharing your home. Especially your mom, who may be uniquely equipped to push your buttons. Debrah's mom came to stay with her for about five weeks before the baby was born and another five weeks after. "It was kind of strained," she says. "Even though it was my only source of adult company, I found it much easier once she was gone. We couldn't really fall into a routine. For ten years I'd lived by myself, and I found it foreign and very stressful to have my home situation be as different as it was."

Sometimes family can surprise you in a positive way, however. Julie was all ready for her conservative mom's visit—straight from the family farm in Manitoba—to be a total nightmare. "I was prepared for a lot of judgment and criticism, and I thought it was going to be hell, but it wasn't," Julie says. Her mom stayed for three weeks when Julie's son Milo was a few months old. Grandma didn't help with baby care, but "having someone always around to talk to—I loved that," Julie says. And when Julie was distraught, having to let Milo occasionally spend the night with Paul, his father and her coparent, having her mom there was invaluable. "We had a great visit, one of the best ever. We bonded a lot."

In fact, bonding with parents seems to be a common by-product of single motherhood. As Kimberley pointed out, for many single moms, their own mother ends up being the closest thing they have to a parenting partner on an emotional level. Even if Grandma lives far away, the grandchild gives mother and adult daughter something to talk about that's important to both of them. It's that way for me. It was a mixed blessing to actually be in the same house as my mom, but now that we're both back in our own spaces I talk to her almost every day, and I'm able to share with her the details no one else wants to hear—like that Scott sat up, stood up, learned how to fake a cough, got a new tooth, climbed the stairs, ate waffles, or bit my arm—and she tells me the details of her day. I've always been in close contact with my mom, but Scott has definitely brought us closer. It's that way for most of the single moms I've talked to. A lovely and unexpected benefit of single motherhood is that it actually builds stronger extended families.

# Infinity and Beyond

*A Peek Into Your*

*Single-Mom Future*

**F**unny thing—the further you get into being a single mother by choice, the less it's about being single and the more it's just about being a mom. Especially after that first postpartum year of adjustment, single mothers have the same things on their minds as any other mothers. Discussions tend to focus on fascinating topics like nursery-school selection, potty-training techniques, and thumb-sucking protocols, not so much on any single-mom-specific struggles. Turns out, single motherhood is just as beautiful to experience and just as potentially boring to talk about as any other kind of motherhood. Yes, some things are just universal. (Even though I do now have a vested interest in these parenting issues, I have to admit I still often tune out these snorefest conversations. Sometimes even when I was the one who initiated them!)

But wait—isn't single motherhood particularly difficult? When some people find out you're a single mom, they look at you like you're brave or crazy or superhuman or all three. "It must be so hard!" But is it really? For me, so far, it's been much easier than I expected it to be. I figured that was mostly good luck. Yet I couldn't get the majority of the single moms I interviewed to go into any detail about trying times. The most I could get from many of them was a chirpy "It's hard—but it's great!" Even the women who had experiences that were objectively really hard—like Laura with her twins and Amanda with her micropreemie—tended to put a positive spin on it. I had to really press them for details. After a while, I had to wonder what was going on. Were these women lying to me? Not wanting to sound like complainers? I hear married and partnered women in my life and in the media talk at length about the difficulty of parenting. What was up with these single moms?

"The single moms who choose to be single moms are a whole different category," explains Charlene, the educational consultant in Chicago who has a four-year-old girl. "Even if things don't work out, you think differently." Indeed, babies born to single moms by choice were so very wanted and their moms, who are usually much older than the typical first-time mom, often had to work so hard to get them that any difficulty is eclipsed by happiness and gratitude.

"When you enjoy it, is it ever really that hard?" asks Melissa, who I spoke to after she'd been up all night with two-month-old twin boys. "Weren't your favorite college classes the ones that were the most challenging?"

"I tried so hard for so long," says Liz, who also has twin boys. "It doesn't feel hard for me, because I'm so happy to have them. I don't ever wake up and feel like I yearn for my old life." Liz lives in a large house in New York City full of modern furniture ("having grown up in a house with tchotchkes all over the place, I tend to go in the opposite direction") with an entire floor just for her sons. "Every morning we meet in the hall and have this huge hugfest, and it feels like every day is like that; we're so happy to see each other."

"I don't have a lot of time to myself," admits Marcy, the navy captain with the two-year-old son, "and sometimes that's hard. But I've gotten used to it, and, honestly, a lot of times I like it 'cause he's fun!"

Whether it's a small stress or a large one, most of the single moms I spoke to seem mature enough to handle it and to have anticipated the hard times, and are determined to put a happy spin on their lives.

How hard parenthood is also depends so much on your temperament and that of the baby, and different stages will be harder or easier for different people. Debrah, whose son is now three, says that having a newborn was the hardest thing she'd ever done. "Even though I'd gone through a surgical residency," she said, "I had never found myself pushed that far before."

Harder than residency? To the best of my understanding, that's pretty much the gold standard of hazing. Besides, she'd already told me she didn't have sleep deprivation as a new mom because the baby slept in bed with her. Isn't sleep deprivation everyone's number one complaint? "Um," I said, trying to phrase it delicately, "what was so hard, exactly?"

"I found myself having to live moment to moment," Debrah answered. "I've always been the type of person who has three-, five-, and ten-year goals." With the baby, she had to downgrade to having a one-day goal of just making it through the day, not knowing exactly what was in store. "This little thing needs you all the time. It was so different for me," she says. She couldn't live the regimented type A life she was used to.

I had to laugh! My sense of time and scheduling is completely compatible with that of an infant. *Having* to live moment to moment? I took to it like a duck to water. It's school age—with its early rising and rigid schedule—that's gonna kick my ass.

How hard it is to parent can also have a lot to do with fear, expectations, and what you're used to. One time after parent-baby yoga class in my yuppie neighborhood, I overheard two married moms saying they'd finally ventured into the subway with their babies alone. Eight months after they were born! Meanwhile, I saw working-class moms navigating the subway alone every day, hefting heavy strollers up and down the many flights of stairs, often keeping other kids in tow as well. Other professional-class moms braved the subway only on weekends, always with husbands to carry the stroller.

Of course, I shouldn't have been so judgmental of those privileged moms for their subway phobia—I'm just as much of a sheltered scaredy-cat as they are in many ways. For me, the big scary thing was navigating Penn Station in Thanksgiving crowds with a five-month-old, a stroller, a backpack, and a giant suitcase. Turns out that when you just suck it up, figure it out, and ask for help, a lot of things are doable. And I think single moms, privileged or not, are more likely to just figure things out, both because they have no choice and because they want a life.

That said, there is a fair amount of sucking it up to be done. Like other single moms by choice, I am so happy to have my baby and I wanted him so badly for so long that any hard times really don't seem so hard. But at least I realized that my perception that single motherhood is easy has partly to do with the degree to which I am psyching myself up for the experience. I went to a cocktail party one Friday night, taking the baby with me (Scott loves a party!). Toward the end of the evening, one of my exes—the one who

wanted kids and who would have made such a great coparent—showed up.
I hadn't seen her in almost two years. Naturally, because she loves children,
she started playing with Scott. After a while, I got my coat, Scott's snowsuit,
my backpack-diaper bag, and the frontpack carrier for Scott, and started the
process of getting us ready to leave.

There was nothing particularly hard about any of it. I was in good spirits, not too tired, not feeling at all burdened by Scott or the impending subway ride home. But as I was juggling the various coats and packs, my ex did
a small, simple thing—she automatically started to help me, closing an open
zipper to my backpack and assisting me with my coat. I don't think it was at
all a conscious act on her part. It was the instinctive behavior of a natural
caretaker. Suddenly it hit me, in a wave of emotion—how hard I was working, how alone I was, and how profoundly easier parenting could be if I had
a supportive partner and coparent doing it with me. So I guess single motherhood *is* hard. Sure, I am aware of the big ways in which it can be hard. But
it took someone making it easier for me in that very small way for me to have
an awareness of how hard single motherhood is in a million other little ways.
As with many other moms I spoke to, the ones I was starting to suspect were
freakish single Stepfords, it doesn't feel so hard in part because I just don't
let myself go there.

## REALITY CHECK

Although most of the moms I interviewed kept up that sunny Stepford
smile about the experience of single motherhood, there were a few
willing to cough up the real deal. "For most people, having a baby is like having a bomb thrown into the center of your life," says Rachel, mom of an
eight-year-old. "My fantasy was, I love children and I just wanted a baby to
hold. I couldn't imagine the major, major life changes I'd go through. Unless you were the oldest in the family or something, you can't imagine it. You
don't know what it's like to be on call 24/7. If you're not watching your
child, you're paying someone to do it. I didn't realize that 'mother' meant
housekeeper, and as a single hipster in San Francisco, it wasn't a priority for
me. But now I'm dealing with a house, laundry, and cooking. With a kid, you
can't just not eat or have a bowl of cereal for dinner.

"It's hard," Rachel adds. "I think we [single moms by choice] just take that as a given. But it's completely worth it."

"The hardest thing for me is probably sleep deprivation," says Carol, whose sixteen-month-old son has just started sleeping through the night. Her sleep problems started at the end of her pregnancy, so "for two years I never got more than four or five hours of sleep at a time," Carol says. "It was affecting my sharpness. I was like, Oh my goodness, could I be getting early Alzheimer's?" Then her son turned out to have multiple food allergies and she had to dramatically change both his diet and the rest of the family's to make sure he didn't ingest something accidentally. "But they're minor things," Carol says cheerily (the woman is so relentlessly upbeat she should become a motivational speaker). "Because you look down the road and he's *going* to sleep through the night," Carol says, "and he'll outgrow most of the food allergies by the time he's two."

"This morning I woke up and I was so tired," says Jessica, mom of thirteen-month-old Ariana. "I got her out of her crib and put her in my bed." Ariana was still restless, so Jessica tried another tack. "Why don't you play with your toys and I'll put a blanket on the floor and watch you and, like, doze." No dice. "I looked at her like, no way are you gonna let me do this." Jessica's exhaustion was painful, she says. "But you know, I had to get over it. I said, OK, I'll get our day going. The way I dealt was to find humor in it. I don't get mad or frustrated or think, This sucks, because that's not fun for her and not fun for me."

"It's hard," agrees Cheri. "The sleep deprivation is hard. And whatever expectations I had, everything's been different. I assumed I'd be having a girl, and I had a boy. I expected the first year to be really hard, I mentally prepared for it, and it wasn't anything like that. Then the second year my son got sick a lot and it was really hard." Still, for Cheri, it all comes out positive.

As upbeat as most single moms are, it is exhausting taking care of a baby and not everyone really wants it or is cut out for it. If you look at it without the rose-colored mommy lenses I almost always seem to wear, it's a physically grueling, nonstop giant hassle. Even the fun stuff can be hard. Here's me frolicking off to an event in Manhattan one very cold day in December with five-and-a-half-month-old Scott: Change baby, bundle up baby in snowsuit and hat, put baby in sling, check to make sure diaper bag has enough diapers, wipes, some toys, and an outfit change just in case. Take extra blanket and professional-quality earmuffs to protect baby's hearing from screeching subway brakes. Uh-oh, look at the time, hurry, hurry, hurry. Put coat, hat, gloves on self. Down three flights of stairs carefully so as not to trip and kill baby, pick up twelve-pound stroller, walk two blocks to subway, get down another flight of stairs with what is now forty pounds of gear (twenty-pound baby, twelve-pound stroller, eight-pound diaper bag). Fumble for wallet. Realize wallet is in another bag back in the apartment. Hurry back up subway stairs, two blocks, three flights to my apartment with twenty-pound baby, get wallet, repeat process. At least the baby wasn't crying, and didn't have one of those poop explosions where you have to strip him and put him in the bathtub! And this was an easy baby—only twenty pounds, still breastfeeding, no formula to prepare, no baby food to bring along. It really helps to be physically strong, and I'm not kidding. I've lifted weights regularly for almost fifteen years and it's a struggle for me sometimes. I don't know how wimpy moms survive. Yes, I choose to live in a third-floor walkup apartment in New York City, so maybe some things are a little harder, but being the primary caretaker of a child is not a walk in the park for any mom, single or otherwise.

Except that it *is* a walk in the park in my experience. Even on bad days, I feel like being a mom isn't very hard. The love and joy balance out the labor and the stress. For me, it lends new meaning to the lyrics "He Ain't Heavy, He's My Brother."

But even with my admittedly easy baby, there are times that are dark. I was pretty worried when Scott got bronchiolitis at about three months and woke up throughout the night coughing his little lungs up, turning red and white and choking on his infected mucus when he wasn't vomiting it up. I was thinking, What if he really chokes in his sleep? What if he can't breathe? I'm a pretty calm mother and these were just fleeting worries, but still. That was nothing, however, compared to the terror I experienced when he had a weird reaction to his six-month vaccines. He woke me up at four in the morning, apparently distressed. I turned on the light and found him hyperactive, manic, his head darting about but his eyes totally vacant. He was feverish and his heart seemed to be racing. He was like one of those drugged-out people you see sometimes on a street corner, crazy smiles on their faces, laughing and rocking and grabbing wildly at invisible flies. I could not get him to focus on me. No one was home. It lasted almost an hour. I took his temperature, gave him Tylenol, and worked myself into a terrible state. I attempted to take his pulse at every vein and artery I knew of (I stupidly didn't know about the artery in the upper arm—the best way to find a pulse in an infant) and couldn't find a consistent pulse. I wondered whether to wake the doctor up for this or be a good girl and end up with a dead kid. Then he went limp and fell asleep. I sure could have used a partner right about then. I called the doctor. She was unconcerned and prescribed Tylenol and "wait and see." So I waited, terrified that he was having seizures that would result in brain damage. Turns out it was probably a REM sleep disturbance. But it scared me to death, and in the middle of the night, I only had old sitcoms to turn to. It's in a crisis, or even a perceived crisis, that single motherhood can really suck.

Indeed, it's not always easy raising a child, especially as a single mom, and the reasons why it's challenging will change over the years as you and the child both grow. "It can be daunting when they're little," says Jane Mattes, whose son is now almost twenty-seven. Being the single mom of an infant can be "physically stressful," she remembers, "and you don't get a lot back emotionally." Then there was a shift, and her son's school-age years were a delight, Jane says, where she "got to watch him become a person." Then another shift: He hit his teen years and became "ornery," she says, and motherhood became quite challenging again. "Your job is *over* now, Mom," her son proclaimed at age sixteen. "That was just the beginning of it," says Jane, who had not expected a hard time from her teenage son, despite all the stories from other parents. "The separation part was hell: letting your children go, and not hanging on too tight, and not pushing them away because they're being so obnoxious. It's hard for any parent, but as a single mom you have to go through letting them go without having someone there to help you keep balanced." Jane's son had good grades, behaved reasonably, and didn't do the things parents most worry about, like drinking and drugs. Still, he went through the typical teen stage of ragging on his mother. "Someone [like a husband] to tell me, 'You're not that bad, dear,' would have been nice," says Jane. But the stage passed—"I think he just grew up; I don't know any other way to put it." But even though she describes her son's teens and early twenties as challenging, Jane says she wouldn't trade the experience of raising him for anything. "It's still absolutely worth it."

## WHAT WILL SINGLE MOTHERHOOD
## DO TO YOUR SOCIAL LIFE?

Grim fact: A lot of single moms by choice end up having little to no adult social life. There are certainly reasons why that's necessary, to some extent, or at least an unavoidable by-product of single parenting. There aren't endless hours in a day, and hopefully you had kids because you actually wanted to spend time with them. When you work all week, leaving your kids with a nanny or in day care or in school, you don't want to turn around and leave the house again without them. Also, you may not have the energy to go out at night or the money to pay a babysitter. But not having a social life ultimately is a choice, and one that the women I spoke to are divided on. Some have basically decided to put their adult social life on a shelf for twenty years, feeling that the kids deserve all their attention. Others, myself included, don't think that's a good idea for either the moms or the kids.

Of course, there are some changes you just can't get around. "Now my social life is pretty much anyone who is willing to come to me and help me with the babies," says Laura, the Brooklyn mother of twin boys. She takes them out to restaurants and the like—"They love it!"—but with two infants, she needs to be out with someone who is willing to pitch in with the baby care.

And some single moms find it difficult to socialize when their contemporaries who have children are all coupled. "The friends I had before Eric was born don't have kids, and the people who do have kids are in couples," says Debrah, the surgeon with the three-year-old son. "I don't think it occurs to people in my social circle that I'm not doing things with other people. You're not really included, because they're all friends by virtue of being couples." Despite some social isolation, Debrah admits, "My life is very full right now. I like what I do, I like my time with my son. I really like being a mother, even more than I thought I would."

"I find I don't really fit in with the married-with-kids crowd," agrees Marcy as well. "The men's wives still see me as a single woman and don't necessarily want me around."

There's a culture clash, any way you slice it, says Charlene. "You've been living in *Sex and the City* with your single girlfriends, and either they have their fantasies [of still finding Prince Charming] or they don't want to deal with children. So you make friends with a lot of couples, but you're left out of certain things because you're not in a couple."

Suzie doesn't have an adult social life and doesn't really miss it. "I go out twice a year without my kids," she says. "I see enough of adults at work. If I was at home it would be different." Suzie says she conducts most of her friendships via e-mails and phone calls. "I have adult companionship. I just don't go *out*. I work and then I go home and play with my kids. We also do neighborhood things so I can have time with adults. I moved into a very family-oriented neighborhood a few years before I had kids. I bought a four-bedroom house, and people were like, 'Uh, Suzie, what?!' " But once she had her kids, the move made a lot of sense.

Of course, the family neighborhood has its downsides. "If there's a neighborhood party without the kids, everybody's married and sometimes that gets a little uncomfortable. Neighbors are always trying to set me up," Suzie reports.

With her focus being so exclusively on the kids, does Suzie worry she'll lose her sense of purpose once the kids grow up and are out of the house? Not really. "I used to volunteer a lot, so I'll probably do more of that."

Like Suzie and many of the women I spoke to, Diana, the single mom of a toddler and a six-year-old, has happily shelved her once-active social life. Her focus has really shifted. "I used to be out every night of the week, but now it's hard to leave at night. Before I had children, I couldn't anticipate what would give, where I would come up with more time. I was really scared about having to give up so much, and sometimes I miss being involved professionally and communally to the degree I was. But that cost seems so small in comparison to the gift of my children. There will be time, later, for me to go to plays and poetry readings and go out dancing," she says. "In the meantime, I'm really, really lucky to have these kids. It just slowly happens that your priorities shift. And it's OK. It's an amazing thing. You get to love and bond with another human being; you get to help them shape their lives and become who they are. It's an incredible privilege."

Jocelyn, who has a fifteen-year-old, has a somewhat balanced social life, but still, much of it revolves around her daughter. "I work and I spend time with my kid and I go to the movies with friends and family. Kids come over to visit and I find them entertaining. A friend of mine from before I had the baby said, 'Oh my God, you don't have a life!' And I thought, no, for the first time I *have* a life. It just wasn't what she considered a life."

## THE IMPORTANCE OF FINDING BALANCE

My first priority is definitely my son, and I think that's as it should be. He comes first, and my life is happily centered on him and his needs. But I think balance and moderation in this is as important as it is in anything else. One of my concerns about single motherhood was the potential to become overly, smotheringly attached to the child, to have the child become so much the focus of your life that neither you nor the child can have a separate identity. Some of the women I spoke to shared that view. "As a single mom, it's so easy just to fall into the feeling that you and the child are 'best friends,' and you can end up using that to prevent the child from moving on," says psychotherapist and single-mom-by-choice Jane Mattes. "It's important to have other meaningful involvements," she says. Being aware of this is key, Jane says, adding that overinvolvement with the child isn't something that just happens with single moms. "It happens to married couples, too," Jane says. Single moms do have particular challenges, though. With just one parent around, the ability to proceed with a personal life can often have a lot to do with money—whether there's enough to hire a babysitter or a housekeeper or other ways to lift the burdens of motherhood so that Mom doesn't have to be on duty every minute. But it isn't entirely about money—it also seems to depend on your attitude, your willingness to be flexible, and the extent to which you actually want a social life.

Sometimes it's the people who love you who prod you to get a life of your own. When Lisa M. had her daughter, "I was so crazy in love with her and she was my every breath," she says. "When she was about eight or nine months old, my mother said, 'You have to go out with your friends,' and I was like, 'Why?'" But with her mom (or other relatives) as a babysitter, Lisa happily found balance and was able to maintain an adult life and date. In fact, she's not actually a single mom anymore—she has found a partner.

With two kids as a single mom, Anne doesn't have a lot of free time. "You can't even compare it to a working job," she says, "because it's every hour of the day or night, feeding, clothing, emotional growth—it's huge." Still, she feels it's essential to carve out a separate life for herself. "If you're raising kids alone, you have to retain some aspect of what makes you happy or you'll go crazy. It might be having a book group or going to the gym or some shred of something that's about you. Take that hot bath, or have that babysitter in once a week, even if it just means going to a café and reading a book. Otherwise, you end up feeling like you're on a treadmill."

Jessica, whose daughter is just over a year old, doesn't feel it's necessary or healthy to abruptly change your life to being totally child-focused. "I've just incorporated her into my life, made some adjustments for her, and it's good!" she says. The nanny comes early, so Jessica can get to the gym, and then she comes home and plays with her daughter before work. Every night, Jessica makes sure she's there to give her daughter a bath and put her to bed, but then she'll often go out with friends. Or she brings her daughter along (something she realizes is the last hurrah of Ariana's infancy—toddlers tend to need more structure and are harder to tote). "My friends and I will go to this place nearby. I'll have her fed and in her little jammies and put her in her stroller and she'll fall asleep. She likes the background noise." Jessica spends a lot of her free time with her daughter, but she also takes breaks and sees babysitters as a positive thing in her daughter's life, not a negative one. "I have a twenty-year-old babysitter on the weekends," Jessica says. "It's great for her. It's a whole new energy, different from me or her nanny."

While many single moms by choice depend on single moms' support groups, Jessica says she's "kind of anti that." Not that she thinks it's a bad thing for others. "I think it's great that it's there, but I don't want to be part of it. I want to integrate. Being a single mom is not something I want to accentuate in my life. And being part of a group would take time away for me. With all that time, I'd rather be doing other things, like trying to find a partner."

Kimberley, pregnant and raising a fourteen-month-old, doesn't have much of a social life right now, outside of work, but she intends to get one again soon, and she feels that's really important. "I don't want my son to ever think my life is about him," she explains. "I want him to feel like he can go out with his friends whether or not I have plans, without worrying that I'm home alone all sad. I think it's important for kids not to have the burden of that. While I love being a mom, it's not at all everything I am. I have to have this other life, because you can't fake that. I think it's kind of pathetic to live through your children."

Kimberley hastens to add that her time with her son is fulfilling, and she wants to make sure they have plenty of family time. "Where I am right now, some people would find boring," she says. But she doesn't find it that way at all. "I work forty hours a week," she says. "It's a social environment and my whole job is to network with people. I don't pack my lunch, because I see that as my time to meet with people I want to see without a baby clinging to me." As a result, Kimberley says, she has tons of friends and opportunities to socialize, and she doesn't feel the need to go out to dinner or parties at night. What she's planning to do more of, though, is go to cultural events. "I'd like to be able to talk to people about the play everyone has seen."

Kimberley went out a lot when her son was an infant, but as he started to get older, she slowed down—partly because he needed a more consistent schedule, but also because she had gone back to a full-time job. "Work kind of puts the kibosh on doing a lot of socializing," she says. "When I get home, I'm tired." And now there's a baby to tend to after work. "I'm used to coming home and having my own life. But when I put my son to bed, I'm not thinking, Oh, I'm missing 60 Minutes! I think, This is what we do right now. If you can't shift your priorities, then this is a hard path."

Still, Kimberley stays connected with friends. Her son is in bed at half past six and sleeps twelve hours straight, so the hours between 6:30 and 10:30 are Kimberley's time to herself. "I clean up the house, pour a glass of wine, and call people."

Liz, who has three-year-old twins, says she has finally reached a point where she's not exhausted, and though as a working mom she wants to maximize her time with the boys, she also makes a point to have personal time scheduled in. "I have a babysitter who stays late once a week, and I try to have [another] babysitter come in once a week." Liz's dedication to life balance is probably a big part of why she's not single anymore but in a happy new relationship.

"Balance is something I'm still working on," says Cheri, whose son is nearly two. "I don't have the energy level, so that holds me back the most. Jack doesn't sleep through the night—there's lots of coughing and checking on him throughout the night, and then I get sick, too." Still, she manages to build in some time for herself, often with the help of her family. "Jack has a really great relationship with my parents. They get Jack time and I get to go to the spa or out with my friends or out on a date."

One of the things that almost all the moms I talked to said about their social life is that, while some old friends fall by the wayside, having a child opens up a whole new world of friendship. "One of the things that has been really nice is joining this community of pregnant women and mothers," says Ellen, mother of two. "I have this new set of friends, people who I wasn't particularly good friends with before, because we have this shared experience."

"It brings different social aspects to your life," says Cheri, in agreement. "Meeting people at the playground, swimming lessons, even people at the grocery store saying hi to Jack. It just opens up new avenues."

## SINGLE MOTHERHOOD'S EFFECT ON YOUR CAREER

Managing the demands of a career and those of a child is hard for any parent, and neither corporate America nor the federal government seems interested in making it any easier. Our system is largely still set up for *Father Knows Best*–style families, where Dad makes the money and Mom stays home. That doesn't work for most married mothers, but for most single moms, there's simply no possibility of staying home. Several women I spoke to were contemplating changing to more flexible, less demanding careers that would be more compatible with single motherhood, though one said being a mom pushed her to find a higher-paying, more "professional" career. Others stay where they are but find themselves switching onto the mommy track, where they have to forgo career advancement in order to maintain a reasonable family life. That's not always the case, though—a few lucky single moms seem to manage to have it all.

Debrah thought that choosing single motherhood—or any kind of motherhood, for that matter—would mean that her surgical career would take a hit. In fact, when she was a resident, she was basically told as much by a female advisor. Since then, however, Debrah has been pleasantly surprised. "The mentors who are men in their fifties have been extremely supportive of me," she says. "They know I'm good at what I do, and that my being a mother doesn't have anything to do with how good a surgeon I am." Yet despite encouraging feedback before the baby came, she still thought actually having a child would have a negative impact on her at work. Not so, she says. "My chair is supportive. No one has stopped asking me to be on committees. In fact, now my boss sends me on seminars about lifestyle and balancing your life, and that wouldn't have been open to me before." Debrah even goes so far as to say she thinks being a mom has improved her skills as a doctor. "I think I'm a better surgeon than I would be if I didn't have Eric," she says. "I'm more tolerant of people, more sensitive. I think it's made me a better person, more empathetic."

Suzie is a director in a financial firm in Tennessee. "I don't have to travel—nowadays people do everything by e-mail and conference calls anyway," she says. "I have a BlackBerry, so I can go on school trips with the kids or to school parties. I go through stressful periods, but it hasn't negatively impacted my career. All the companies I've worked for have been supportive, because they know I'll get the job done. I think you just have to have a balance and find the right company." That doesn't mean you can literally have it all, though, Suzie says. "Sometimes I can't take on a project at work or I can't pick up the kids at choir practice every day. But I do get home at quarter past five every day and we have a family dinner and have breakfast in the morning." Though she has been successful at work, she has had to take the mommy track occasionally. "I have given up promotions. Like right now, my boss is waiting to retire until I'm ready to take over from him. But I have to think about it. For a period of time it'll be more hours. Is it worth it to give up the extra time with the kids?"

Alice decided to have a kid even though she says, "I knew I was probably hurting my career." And has it? She has retained her high-paying job as a telecommunications executive, but she feels she has hit, if not a glass ceiling, a sippy-cup ceiling. "Some may have thought my choosing to be a single mom was morally inappropriate," Alice guesses. But she thinks the ceiling has more to do with paternalistic assumptions about what her priorities are going to be, or should be: "Well, now she's a single mom so she can't be the kind of businesswoman she was; we will not give her the same opportunities." Alice had anticipated this line of thinking, so before she had her son, she sat down with her boss and said, "Look, don't leave me out of things because you think I can't do it because of my parental responsibilities. Let me decide." Still, in the end, Alice says, her bosses have done the deciding for her. Despite the career slowdown, she wouldn't change anything. "The net-net is clearly positive," she says, sounding more boardroom than playroom. "It is not a chore, it's a pleasure to be with him. Do I get tired or frustrated? Yes. But it's a joy."

Seniority can smooth out some work issues—one plus to being an older mom. "I'm lucky that I'm senior enough that if I have to take a day off from work because my son's sick, I take the day off, and the world's not coming to an end," says Marcy, who is a captain in the navy.

Erron, the medical resident, thinks having a baby may actually be making work-life balance a little more manageable. "Some of the other residents are more stressed," she reports. "I think it's easier for me to get home and leave work behind. No matter how bad things are at work, I come home and here's this little boy smiling from ear to ear, and that makes me so happy."

And for some women, a mommy-track attitude can be a healthy thing. Melissa, the mom of infant twins, feels like having kids has created a positive, empowering shift for her in the workplace. "I was always trying to be the good girl, to smooth things over, be the person at work who always stays late, who's always available," she explains—"and now I'm not!" Like Melissa, when I have worked in an office, I have tended to be that perfectionistic person who always stays late, getting to be pals with the midnight office-cleaning staff. All that changed the instant I had Scott. His needs and my desire to be with him and to take care of myself so that I can be in good emotional and physical shape for him literally enforce balance in my life and work, and that has been a wonderful thing.

## HAVING MORE THAN ONE CHILD

The minute I had Scott, literally that week, when I was extremely weak from loss of blood and practically still had the IVs in my arm, people started asking me, "So you gonna have a second one?"

Good question, is my best answer. Like many of the single moms I spoke to, I always envisioned having more than one kid. I thought for sure I'd have two and I'd love to have a sibling for Scott. I grew up with three siblings and can't imagine life as an only child. But for me, the idea of raising two kids alone seems daunting, both logistically and financially. I am sure I could do it and it would work out fine. But without family in town, I'd be even more dependent than I am now on either friends or hired help to back me up in a pinch. I'm not comfortable imposing on nonfamily to that extent, and I don't see myself making enough money to have round-the-clock hired help available. Also, friends who are parents have told me that you can take one child with you to a lot of places. Add another child and you have to stay home. As a single parent, that could get really isolating.

I'm still thinking about it, though. Every time I go to the Tea Lounge, a major new-mom hangout in my neighborhood, I look at the brand-new babies and I am filled with longing. I do have twelve vials of my donor's sperm sitting in cold storage (at three hundred and thirty dollars per year), waiting to help me create a full sibling for Scott, so if my aging eggs were willing to cooperate, I could do it. We'll see.

I'm not the only single mom thinking about having another, and a few women I talked to have already done just that.

"Having the second, I felt fear similar to when I was thinking about having the first," says Diana, whose children are one and six. "It was a huge leap of faith. I think having a child is about the most terrifying endeavor you can embark on. You never know what will come out—temperament, personality, abilities, disabilities—you just have no clue." For Diana, having two has been both a challenge and a joy. "People say it's not double but triple the work. Let's just say it's a lot of work—mental, physical, emotional, logistical—but I'm managing, and learning more than I ever knew I would about myself as well as about parenting. It's amazing to have a second child. It makes us feel more like a family than a pair. And my daughter is so grateful to have her younger brother. She's an incredible sister and it's joyful to see that part of her, which I would not have known otherwise."

A lot of women feel, as Diana does, that three makes a "real" family. Kimberley, who is currently pregnant with her second child, says, "For me, having just the two of us at Christmas is kind of like having a bare lightbulb hanging down from the middle of the apartment."

"Having a second child took more thought," says Ellen, "because I'd had the first and knew how hard it was. I didn't necessarily want another baby, but I wanted my daughter to have a sibling." With Ellen, as with a lot of single moms by choice who end up having more than one kid, the desire was based in her appreciation for her own sibling. Ellen has a brother, and while they don't talk all the time, "I really appreciate being able to call him and say, 'You'll never guess what Mom just said; she's crazy!' Or just to share memories." Having a second child was also a way for Ellen to help her child feel less alone and less unusual. "I live in a neighborhood where everyone is married heterosexual parents," Ellen says. As a family headed by a single, straight mom, she and her daughter didn't fit in perfectly. "One thing I can give her is a sibling," Ellen reasoned. Her parents were mixed in their reaction to the idea. "Dad said, 'Have another!'" Ellen remembers. But her mom was much more cautious, telling Ellen, "Think about this. You're already so tired." Financially, it has been much more of a burden and a risk, Ellen says. "Paying for two in day care means that once the two of them are in public school I will have no savings left."

"I'm very close to my sister. I've got a special relationship with her, and I wanted to have that for Christina," says Suzie. "It was a hard two years until Eliza was about two, but now it's so much easier to have two. They're so close, they like to play together. They occupy each other."

Lisa M. always thought she'd have more than one kid, but first she had to be ready—when you have one child, she says, "you never think you could have that kind of love in your heart, in your body, in your soul, for anybody else." Then, she felt her daughter had to be ready. When her daughter was younger, Lisa says, "I'd ask, 'Do you want Mommy to have a brother for you?' And she was like, 'Uh, I'd like a turtle.' So she wasn't ready. Then when she was seven, I asked again and she said, 'Yes, that would be cool!' " By that time Lisa was in her late thirties and knew her insurance wouldn't cover the in vitro fertilization process she needed because of her damaged fallopian tubes. Also, she really wanted a son. "Within the week, I called the adoption agency."

Adopting her son was a very different process than the one she went through to have her daughter. "The insemination, the IVF, that was me deciding what I was going to do for my life," Lisa remembers. With adoption, someone else was making the decisions as to whether she'd be a fit parent. "It wasn't a private adoption where I had all this money to basically buy a child," she says. "It was through the foster-care system here. I felt like I was under this microscope." The home-study process was long and involved—it took more than two years—but "once they did the match, it was like wildfire." Her future son was a thirteen-month-old boy named Kanye who had been with a foster family since birth.

"Meeting him, he was such a cool soul," Lisa says. "I'd go and visit him every day, and within three weeks he was in our home. He's only been here for three or four months, but it seems like he's always been here. It's so fulfilling. I feel like I get it now. I'm more part of the team. Everybody in my family's got two or three kids. I've got my family now." Having gone through so much trouble to bear a biological child, does she feel any differently about Kanye than about Mariah, the daughter she birthed? "I love them the same," says Lisa. "You hear it, but you don't understand it till you're in it. The adopted kids are born from your heart, and that's how I feel."

Of course, sometimes having two kids—or more—happens in one fell swoop, especially for older single moms who used fertility drugs. For Liz, who has twins, the shock of having two has morphed into appreciation. "It's great watching them together," she says. "I can't fathom having one kid now. The dynamic of the two of them is my favorite part of being a mom."

## HAPPY ENDINGS

So has your life totally changed?" people always ask. I guess so, though I have to say it doesn't feel like it. I'm the same person, and I wanted this baby so much that to me, the changes don't seem as radical as they really are. Sure, I'm a little thicker around the middle than I used to be. I probably won't go out to the movies for the next ten years, since without Scott it's fifty dollars to leave the house and I'd just as soon wait for a film to come out on DVD. I'm a lot less likely to spend money on things I don't need. Or even on things I do need—I've never been much of a shopper, but with a baby in tow shopping is not always the most enjoyable of activities, especially when you don't have a car to transport the goods back home. I guess there are some emotional changes, too. I've always been sentimental, but now it's sentimentality on overdrive. Can I blame it on postpartum hormones that when I exited the Times Square subway station with almost-six-month-old Scott and he began to look around at all the neon, I started to tear up: "His first trip to Times Square!" Are there even any hormones *left* six months after giving birth? Or am I doomed to be one of those embarrassing sentimental moms who has to always carry a hanky? The biggest change, though, is how happy I am. I didn't feel unhappy before. But people who haven't seen me since the baby was born remark on it. *Happy, relaxed, content* are the kinds of words they use. And I am. I have a family at last.

Most other single moms seem to feel the same. "I'm just so happy on a daily basis," reports Carol, whose youngest boy is sixteen months old. "I look at my son and think, you may wear me out but I'm so glad I have you." Seeing the world through the eyes of a toddler is such a treat, Carol says. Even dull errands become adventures. "You take him to the mall and, whoa, his eyes are like buckets, just walking through the plaza."

Marcy agrees. "Being a mom has been everything I had hoped for," she says, "and I have absolutely no regrets. My son is now in the throes of his terrible twos, but even with all that, I still love being a mom."

Even though it's hard, says Anne, who is raising two children on her own, "something about having kids really galvanizes you. You feel empowered." Empowerment was a theme echoed by other women who have chosen to be moms, like Melissa, the single mother of twins. "I feel empowered that I went ahead and did the one thing I really wanted to do. I look at my sons and feel I am truly the luckiest woman on earth."

"I am truly better for having become a mom," says Debrah. "It gives you a sense that there's more important things to life than what you are doing right now. I love going home and watching this little person suck up knowledge. Here's someone who is relying on you for not only the necessities in life but also for entertainment and love and whatever you might give them. I don't know if I ever really thought about how it would be. I never had to *decide* whether or not to have children; for me, it was more of an instinct. But I find it a lot more entertaining, more fun, more full of joy than I thought it would be. If I had to die tomorrow so that this child would live, I would have no problem with that. It's harder than you think it's going to be, but it's also easier than you think it's going to be," Debrah says. "I don't know that I would have chosen to do it any differently than I'm doing it now because I've had such a good time."

All the single moms I talked to, even the non-Stepford types, tend to gush when they talk about the rewards of motherhood. "It's such a unique experience," says Cheri, mom of a two-year-old. "I wasn't prepared for how amazing it would be in all aspects. To me, he's just this little miracle," she gushes, "and I know women give birth a million times a day."

"It's been hard and scary," says Shannon, whose daughter is now two, "but when I look at my daughter, I know I did the right thing. She's beautiful, precious, fun-loving, and winds people around her little fingers wherever she goes."

Lisa M. says her two kids give real purpose to her life. "I used to think there's no such thing as forever until I had my daughter," Lisa says, "and she's my forever. She's the one thing and the one person who will always be there, and I'll always be there for her. She's my solid ground. And when I adopted my son, it was just more so."

"For the most part, I've been deliriously happy since I had her," says

Jocelyn, the psychologist from Phoenix who has the fifteen-year-old daughter. "Everything else was just filler."

As I finish this book, Scott is nine months old and he's more of a challenge every day. He's standing, walking holding on, crawling at warp speed, climbing stairs, and getting into everything, especially if it's dangerous—the stairs, the stove, the fireplace, the toilet, plastic bags, electrical cords. I can't leave him unsupervised for a moment. He's developing quite a strong will of his own, and I wonder how terrible those twos will be—even now when he doesn't get his way he sometimes throws a fit. We have daily arguments regarding whether or not the toilet bolt cover is a toy. Every day I say no. Every day he lets me know, often in a heartrending Oscar-worthy performance, that I'm the meanest mom in the world for not letting him play with it. He's more of a handful, but at the same time with every passing day he's more of a companion and he brings me more joy with the joy he finds in everything. The playground. A leaf. A balloon. A funny face that I made. The person sitting next to us on the subway. He's a gregarious little guy, charming and flirting with everyone in sight, batting his big blue-gray eyes, laughing out loud, loving life and making everyone around him love it, too. And there's something new. Just the other day, I came through the door after working at the Tea Lounge for a few hours, and Scott saw I was home. "It's Mommy!" the nanny told him. Scott took off and headed straight for me as fast as he could, as if his life depended on it, his little hands stomping across the floor, elbows bowed like a bulldog's, his head down so he could make better time. "Ma ma ma ma ma ma ma!!!" he cried for the first time ever as he raced toward me. I scooped him up and hugged him tight. "Ma ma ma!" he said, voice muffled, face pressed into my neck as he hugged me back. I don't think I've ever heard a more beautiful sound.

The love affair doesn't end with infancy. It's been twenty-six years since Jane Mattes's baby was born, and she's as full of love as she ever was. "When I get together with my son now," she says, "my heart sings for days."

I think Anne, the northern California single mom who has two kids, said it best: "If you know you want to have a child, you won't regret it. Even though it'll be a huge lifestyle change and you'll make limitless sacrifices, you will have a love that's like no other love you have ever experienced. I can't even put it into words."

# Acknowledgments

This book would never have been written if it weren't for three people and a lot of dumb luck. Molly Manning encouraged me to shelve my self-loathing and take writing classes just for the deadlines they'd impose, even though I thought that was lame and that I should develop self-discipline somehow, instead. One class I took as a result was the amazing Sue Shapiro's one-day Mediabistro memoir workshop. One of her guest speakers that day was Ryan Fischer-Harbage, then an editor at Simon & Schuster. During the twenty minutes Ryan was there, Sue happened to choose the first page of my memoir about my 1996 brain injury to read aloud, from her stack of forty student papers. Ryan liked it enough to contact me the next day. Months later he learned I was pregnant as a single mother by choice, and he suggested I write a book on the topic. A couple of months after that, Ryan quit editing, became my agent, and sold the proposal I'd written based on his suggestion—less than a week after I gave birth to Scott. Was I lucky or what?

Many thanks to my editor, Lucia Watson, who bought the idea and was incredibly patient about it when I turned the manuscript in two months late, and to publicist Anne Kosmoski for spreading the word. Then a giant thank-you to Jennie Livingston, who read my rough draft and made lots of excellent critiques—I wish I had been able to do everything she suggested, but I would have blown my deadline by several more months if I had! Thanks also to Joan Hilty, Shoshana Kerewsky, Rachel Pepper, and Akiba Solomon, who all gave me substantive comments. Other readers who also helped me be less clueless were Diane Penn, Martha Willoughby,

Susanna Stein, Rose Arce, Katie Taylor, and Melissa McCoy. Jeannie Kim read the proposal and gave me edits and encouragement. Thanks also to Sally Gardner, Laura Perry, Jeff Bond, Joni Jensen, Navah Steiner, Gerd Grace, Dana Monello, Wendy Dembo, Lucy Mackerras, and Nanette Gartrell for reading the manuscript and being a cheering section. Nina Herzog and Carole Zimmer critiqued early bits, encouraged me, and were very kind in welcoming Scott as the newest member of our writers' group. Thanks to Ximena Bernal for being such a terrific nanny, and to my auxiliary babysitters Gloria Winter and Lucy Shapiro—I wouldn't have got any writing done without you. Kevin Creedon cooked me dinner a million times, and he and Jeff allowed Scott and me to have a lot of fun every Tuesday night. Sally kept me entertained and plied me with passion-fruit martinis. Thanks to all the guys (and gals) from Frim Fram who were willing to Lindy Hop with a pregnant lady—especially Chris Vongsawat and JamieSue Clark—and much love to Elena Ianucci and Joe Palmer and all the folks at Dance Manhattan for letting Scott continue to dance with me even after he was born! *Namaste* to Trish Fox at Park Slope Yoga Center for keeping me in decent shape over the past year and being such a fan of my little "Ambassador of Love." Thanks to my support system: my wonderful family—Mom, Edward, Isabel, and Caroline—and all my friends, especially Susanna, Melodie Winawer, Sally, Kevin, Jeff, Rose, Maria Rueda, Amy Leidtke, Karen Holler, Brad Miskell, Jennie, Mae, Susan Rittscher, Anne Mollegen Smith, David Smith, Amanda Smith, Melissa Cook, Joni, Katie, Maryellen Ward, Joan, Nancy Goldstein, Carolyn Kramer, Julie Friesen, Leanh Nguyen, Roberta Franzheim, Joy Makon, Tom Lowe, Jane Sasseen, Nina Jacobson, Ed Stein, Steve Lin, Cathy Renna, Leah McElrath, and Rachel Pickus. Much gratitude to Charlie Harris for making me soup when I was really sick, and to Jared Keel for hauling the world's heaviest suitcase up the stairs for me. Thanks to Jackie Woodson, Linda Villarosa, Nell Bernstein, Dave Shenk, and Megan McAndrew for writerly advice. And thanks to my doctors: Marianne Legato, for telling me to hurry up; Amalia Kelly (and partners Cristina Matera and Maureen Moomjy), for knocking me up; Sharon Patrick, for shepherding me through most of my pregnancy; and Juanita Jenyons and Allegra Cummings, for delivering Scott safely. Thanks to Veronica Barrios, formerly of Pacific Reproductive Services, for making a stressful process much, much more pleasant. Thanks to Jada Shapiro, for being a fabulous doula, childbirth instructor, and birth photographer. Thanks to Joanna Scheib and Susan Golombok, for sending me copies of academic studies. And thanks to Claire Cavanah, Beth Cramer, Carlos Chiossone, John Stoltenberg, Heidi Ernst, Emily Lewis, Julie Tupler of Maternal Fitness, Hernán Merea, Carolyn Pallof, Arlyn Gajilan, Jason Priest, Bill, Jon Kiehnau, Arthur Fried,

Jennifer Hatch, Cindra Feuer, Basia Hellwig, Donna Minkowitz, Sharon Morris, Carol Simons, Victoria Shah, Simone Leigh, Deborah Apton, Melia Patria, Jennifer Hershey, Jennifer Bergstrom, Constance Costas, Yoonski Lee, and Betsey Biggs. Gold stars for random acts of kindness in times of need go to Tom Sawyer and to Christy Prunier Doss and David Doss. Thanks to Susan Heroy, Joan Griffith, and Shelley Barth for teaching me and encouraging me to write.

Thanks to Jane Mattes of Single Mothers by Choice for allowing me to mine her membership for stories. Most of all, thanks to the many inspiring women who agreed to be interviewed for this book. What a gift to be able to spend the first few months of my postpartum working life talking to you! I hope I have told your stories well. There were times when I was holding a breast-feeding infant with one hand while taking notes with the other, the phone wedged between my shoulder and ear. I think I still got everything down right, but if I made any mistakes, I hope you will forgive me!

# Donor Insemination and Fertility Glossary

*There are lots more terms, but here are the ones used in this book.*

**Anonymous sperm donor:** A man who has donated sperm at a sperm bank. Offspring never have access to the identity of the donor, unless he has agreed to be an open-identity donor.

**Artificial insemination:** Using anything other than a penis to place semen or sperm in the vagina or uterus. Usually a needleless syringe is used, and sometimes also a catheter. Turkey basters don't actually work as well—too big!

**Assisted reproductive technology:** Any medical procedure (like IUI or IVF) used to achieve conception without sexual intercourse.

**Basal body temperature:** Your lowest daily body temperature, taken first thing in the morning. The basal temperature fluctuates throughout a woman's cycle and can help predict ovulation—helpful for timing inseminations. Charting your temperature can help with home inseminations, and some fertility doctors ask patients to do it (others rely on blood tests and ultrasounds to determine ovulation).

**Beta hCG test:** A blood test for hCG, the pregnancy hormone. Can detect a very early pregnancy and help indicate whether an early pregnancy is progressing normally.

**Catheter:** A soft plastic tube, used in artificial insemination to extend the reach of a syringe, allowing sperm to be deposited close to the cervix or into the uterus.

**Cervical mucus:** The mucus seen on the cervix changes throughout a woman's cycle and can help predict ovulation—helpful for timing home inseminations. That's why one woman was reading a pamphlet called "Get to Know Your Cervix."

**Charting:** See basal body temperature.

**Follicle:** A fluid-filled sac containing an egg about to be released.

**Follicle stimulating hormone (FSH):** The level of this hormone present on day three of a woman's menstrual cycle is used as a predictor of the quality and quantity of a woman's eggs. Levels under 10 are considered good; the lower the better.

**Gamete:** A reproductive cell. In women, eggs; in men, sperm.

**Human chorionic gonadotropin (hCG):** The hormone produced in early pregnancy. Also used via injection to trigger ovulation.

**Hysterosalpingogram (HSG):** An X-ray of the pelvic organs in which dye is injected through the cervix into the uterus and fallopian tubes. This test checks for malformations of the uterus and blockage of the fallopian tubes.

**Identity-release donor:** Trademarked term for open-identity donors at the Sperm Bank of California, which pioneered open donors. See open-identity donor.

**Intracervical insemination (ICI):** Placing semen in the vagina using a syringe or a syringe and catheter (the turkey baster method).

**Intrauterine insemination (IUI):** Placing "washed" sperm (semen is removed) in the uterus using a long, thin catheter and a syringe.

**In vitro fertilization (IVF):** Patient takes fertility drugs that cause her to produce multiple eggs. They are harvested (minor surgery) and fertilized outside the body. One or more embryos (usually two or three) are then placed in the uterus. Any additional embryos can be frozen for later use.

**Liquid nitrogen:** A supercold gas used to store and transport frozen semen.

**Open-identity donor:** A sperm donor who agreed, when he donated, that the sperm bank can release identifying information to any offspring who request it when they turn eighteen. Usually he has agreed to at least a one-time contact with any biological children.

**Reproductive endocrinologist:** A gynecologist who specializes in fertility.

**"Washed" sperm:** Sperm that has been separated from the semen, which is replaced with another liquid. Semen, which is normally filtered out by the cervical mucus, irritates the uterus, so it is removed in order to perform an intrauterine insemination.

**"Yes" donor:** See open-identity donor.

# Resources

## BOOKS

*Means really great books that you might not think to get but should.*

### If you only read a few books:
### Guidebooks on choosing single motherhood

*Choosing Single Motherhood: The Thinking Woman's Guide*
Mikki Morrissette • Minneapolis, Be-Mondo Publishing, 2005
Comprehensive how-to by a single mom and former magazine editor.

*Single Mothers by Choice: A Guidebook for Single Women Who Are Considering or Have Chosen Motherhood*
Jane Mattes, CSW • New York, Three Rivers Press, 1994, updated 1997
    The classic guide, still quite relevant, written by a psychotherapist and single mom. Good psychological advice.

### A great read (that's also educational)

*Buying Dad: One Woman's Search for the Perfect Sperm Donor**
Harlyn Aizley • Los Angeles, Alyson Publications, 2003

This book was a best seller. It's a terrific memoir, funny and touching, so well written that it should appeal to anyone—gay, straight, male, female—whether or not they're interested in donor insemination. It's by a partnered lesbian about her personal journey, from the search for sperm to fears of infertility and finally to the birth of her daughter. It will give you a great idea of what the whole process is like.

## Other books I'd recommend:
### Advice for donor-conceived families

*Mommies, Daddies, Donors, Surrogates: Answering Tough Questions and Building Strong Families*
Diane Ehrensaft, Ph.D.  •  New York, Guilford Press, 2005
This excellent book covers how you might feel about using a donor, how to talk about donor-insemination with your child and others, and discusses how the children of assisted reproductive technology fare psychologically. Written by a psychologist. Highly recommended.

### Getting pregnant through donor insemination

*The New Essential Guide to Lesbian Conception, Pregnancy & Birth*
Stephanie Brill  •  Los Angeles, Alyson Books, 2006
Obviously, this is aimed at lesbians, but it has much to offer straight single women, and it openly states that in its introduction. It's a comprehensive book, written by a midwife, and covers all aspects of fertility and donor insemination. It includes sample known-donor legal agreements and coparenting agreements.

*The Ultimate Guide to Pregnancy for Lesbians: How to Stay Sane and Care for Yourself from Preconception Through Birth*
Rachel Pepper  •  San Francisco, Cleis Press, 2005
Written by a lesbian who is a single mom by choice, this guidebook covers fertility and donor insemination in a more personal and engaging way. Though aimed primarily at lesbians, it's inclusive of straight single women.

*Helping the Stork: The Choices and Challenges of Donor Insemination*
Carol Frost Vercollone, MSW, Heidi Moss, MSW, and Robert Moss, Ph.D.  •  Hoboken, NJ, Wiley Publishing, Inc., 1997
This book is mainly for infertile heterosexual couples, though the authors hope

single women and lesbian couples will overlook the emphasis on couples and trans-late the information to suit their needs. Good information, though there's a lot of focus on secrecy and shame issues that may not be relevant to single moms by choice.

### Research on single-mother families

*Raising Boys Without Men: How Maverick Moms Are Creating
the Next Generation of Exceptional Men*
Peggy Drexler, Ph.D., with Linden Gross • Emmaus, PA, Rodale Press, 2005
Written by a (straight, married) Cornell psychology professor and based on her study of single and lesbian moms who are raising boys. Well written, reassuring, and empowering.

*Single by Chance, Mothers by Choice: How Women Are Choosing Parenthood
Without Marriage and Creating the New American Family*
Rosanna Hertz • New York, Oxford University Press, 2006
A slightly dense but still readable book written by a Wellesley sociology profes-sor. Interviews with sixty-five single moms by choice, placed in a sociological and historical context. Useful information, insights, and ideas in a more academic package.

### General pregnancy and childbirth

*What to Expect When You're Expecting*
Heidi Murkoff, Arlene Eisenberg, and Sandee Hathaway, BSN • New York,
Workman, 1984, updated 2002
The classic guidebook. Some find it to be a bit alarmist (lots about what might go wrong), but I just found it to be comprehensive.

*The Pregnancy Book: Month by Month, Everything You Need to Know
from America's Baby Experts* and *The Birth Book: Everything You Need
to Know to Have a Safe and Satisfying Birth*
William Sears, M.D., and Martha Sears, R.N. • New York, Little, Brown and
Company, 1997 and 1994
Good general guidebooks, slightly less comprehensive but more reassuring. Bal-anced information, though the Searses themselves tend toward the natural and progressive.

*The Girlfriends' Guide to Pregnancy: Or Everything Your Doctor Won't Tell You*
Vicki Iovine • New York, Pocket Books, 1995
A funny, friendly guide with advice like your friends are lying when they tell you that you look more beautiful than ever while pregnant. She's got some opinions that are opposite mine—like she's antiexercise and pro–C-section—but it's an enjoyable and informative read.

*Ina May's Guide to Childbirth*
Ina May Gaskin • New York, Bantam, 2003
An inspirational and practical guide written by a well-known Tennessee-based midwife. It will open your mind to the possibility that labor and childbirth can actually be enjoyable. Bonus: a photograph of a woman having an ecstatic (read: orgasmic) delivery. Wow!

*Baby Catcher: Chronicles of a Modern Midwife\**
Peggy Vincent • New York, Scribner, 2003
Engaging and funny account of the author's experiences doing hospital and home deliveries as a labor-and-delivery nurse and then as a midwife, and how it transformed her ideas about how childbirth is managed in this country. A really great read. Highly recommended.

### Taking care of a baby

*Operating Instructions: A Journal of My Son's First Year\**
Anne Lamott • New York, Ballantine, 1993
This was a best seller, for good reason. Lamott got pregnant by accident at thirty-five. Her boyfriend took off immediately, and she decided to have the baby as a single mom. This is her hilarious, startlingly honest, totally engaging account of her son's infancy. A reality check for prospective single moms—she doesn't have an easy time of it—but also a good laugh and a great read.

*Our Babies, Ourselves: How Biology and Culture Shape the Way We Parent\**
Meredith F. Small • New York, Anchor Books, 1998
An engagingly written, well-researched book by a Cornell University anthropologist. Looks at infant-rearing practices from historical, medical, biological, and cross-cultural perspectives. Fascinating and reassuring. Not a how-to book, though it will help inform your thinking about a variety of parenting practices. Highly recommended.

*The Baby Book: Everything You Need to Know About Your Baby*
*from Birth to Age Two*
William Sears, M.D., and Martha Sears, R.N. • New York, Little, Brown and
Company, 1992, updated 2003
Comprehensive and reassuring guidebook by a Harvard-trained pediatrician and
his wife, who is a nurse. They have eight children of their own, so their advice
comes from extensive experience on all fronts. Covers child development, health
care, breast-feeding, sleep issues, and first aid. Includes useful stuff like recommended
doses of over-the-counter medications for infants. They have a more progressive approach to parenting, but the book has much to offer even if you don't follow their
parenting advice.

*What to Expect the First Year*
Arlene Eisenberg, Heidi Murkoff, and Sandee Hathaway, BSN • New York,
Workman, 1989, updated 2003
A good all-around guidebook. Includes a variety of parenting approaches, from
traditional to progressive.

*The Happiest Baby on the Block: The New Way to Calm Crying*
*and Help Your Newborn Baby Sleep Longer*
Harvey Karp, M.D. • New York, Bantam, 2002
This book is about soothing newborns, and I didn't get it till my son was nearly
six months old. But as it turned out, I had used a lot of the techniques in the book,
and they worked quite well for me!

### General readings on motherhood that might help inform your choice

*Mothers Who Think: Tales of Real-life Parenthood*
Camille Peri and Kate Moses, eds. • New York, Washington Square Press
Essays, 1999
Essays on motherhood by more than thirty women writers, from Salon.com.

*Maybe Baby: 28 Writers Tell the Truth About Skepticism, Infertility, Baby Lust,*
*Childlessness, Ambivalence, and How They Made the Biggest Decision of*
*Their Lives*
Lori Leibovich, ed. • New York, HarperCollins, 2006
Essays on the decision, divided into three sections: No Thanks, Not for Me; On
the Fence; and Taking the Leap.

*The Bitch in the House: 26 Women Tell the Truth About Sex, Solitude, Work,*
*Motherhood, and Marriage*
Cathi Hanauer, ed. • New York, Perennial, 2002

*The Bastard on the Couch: 27 Men Try Really Hard to Explain*
*Their Feelings About Love, Loss, Fatherhood, and Freedom*
Daniel Jones, ed. • New York, Perennial Currents, 2004
These great essays on parenting and relationships might help you feel grateful
that you're single! The editors are married to each other.

*Perfect Madness: Motherhood in the Age of Anxiety*
Judith Warner • New York, Riverhead Books, 2005
A best-selling manifesto about contemporary motherhood. May strike a chord if
you're a type A perfectionist (or think you should be).

## ACADEMIC STUDIES ON SINGLE MOTHERHOOD
## AND DONOR-CONCEIVED CHILDREN

I have selected a few of the most relevant studies and summarized their findings.

"Children Raised in Fatherless Families from Infancy: A Follow-up of
Children of Lesbian and Single Heterosexual Mothers at Early Adolescence"
Fiona MacCallum and Susan Golombok, Family and Child Psychology
Research Centre, City University, London • published in *Journal of Child*
*Psychology and Psychiatry* 45:8 (2004), pp. 1,407–1,419
**Salient findings:** Children had more interaction with their moms than kids in
father-present families, but also more conflict, since mom does all the disciplining.
No negative effects on social and emotional development were found due to the absence of a father. Boys in single-mom families had more "feminine" qualities—like
being sensitive and caring—but no fewer masculine qualities than boys in families
with fathers present. There was no evidence that the moms' sexual orientation had
any influence on the socioemotional development of the children.

"Psychosocial Adjustment Among Children Conceived via Donor
Insemination by Lesbian and Heterosexual Mothers"
R. W. Chan, B. Raboy, and C. J. Patterson, University of Virginia • published
in *Child Development* 69 (1998), pp. 443–457

**Salient findings:** In this study of eighty families living in twenty-two states, both parents and teachers reported that the children are well adjusted, socially competent, and exhibiting no unusual behavior problems. Children's well-being was found to be more a function of parenting and relationships within the family than whether the households were headed by a single mother, a heterosexual couple, or a lesbian couple.

"The National Lesbian Family Study 4: Interviews with Ten-Year-Old Children"
Nanette Gartrell, M.D., Carla Rodas, MPH, Amalia Deck, MSN, Heidi Peyser, M.A., Amy Banks, M.D. • published in *American Journal of Orthopsychiatry* 7:4 (October 2005), study available on the Web at www.nllfs.org

**Salient findings:** This is part of a longitudinal study (since 1986) of seventy-eight families of lesbian couples and single lesbian moms. All the kids are donor-conceived. Some have known donors and others have anonymous donors. In social and psychological development, the kids were comparable to children raised in heterosexual families, though the girls in the study demonstrated fewer behavioral problems than their peers in heterosexual families. There was no difference in psychological functioning in children with known donors versus those with unknown donors. Although the children with known donors benefited from having a father, according to their mothers, most who had not yet met or would never meet their donor were unconcerned about not having a father. The children who can eventually meet their anonymous donors were nearly evenly divided in regretting that they had to wait until they were eighteen and in not caring about the prospective meeting. Seventy percent of children with permanently unknown donors had no regrets about not having a father. According to lead researcher Gartrell, for those kids who did have regrets, they characterized those regrets as mild.

"Single Parenthood, Achievement, and Problem Behavior in White, Black, and Hispanic Children"
Henry N. Ricciuti, Ph.D., Department of Human Development, College of Human Ecology, Cornell University • published in the *Journal of Educational Research* 97:4, pp. 196–206

**Salient findings:** This study of almost fifteen hundred twelve- and thirteen-year-old children found little or no evidence of systematic negative effects of single parenthood on children's academic performance or behavior. What mattered most to the kids' outcomes was the mother's education and ability level, regardless of her income or ethnicity. Ricciuti stated that his findings suggest that when the mother is educated, has "positive child expectations," and access to social resources supportive of parenting, single motherhood in itself need not be a risk factor for academic or behavior problems.

"Adolescents with Open-Identity Sperm Donors:
Reports from 12- to 17-year-olds"
J. E. Scheib, M. Riordan, and S. Rubin
The lead researcher, Scheib, is at the Department of Psychology, University of California, Davis • published in *Human Reproduction* 20:1 (2005), pp. 239–252

**Salient findings:** The majority of kids felt comfortable with their donor-insemination origins. Most were curious about the donor and planned to contact him at some point, though not necessarily at age eighteen. Few described him as being an important person in their lives. Most wanted to know what he is like in order to know more about themselves. Most kids were interested in contacting and meeting - half siblings.

"Choosing Identity-Release Sperm Donors: The Parents' Perspective 13–18 Years Later"
J. E. Scheib, M. Riordan, and S. Rubin
The lead researcher, Scheib, is at the Department of Psychology, University of California, Davis • published in *Human Reproduction* 18:5 (2003), pp. 1,115–1,127

**Salient findings:** Almost no parents regretted choosing an open-identity donor. The children were told about their donor-insemination conception from an early age and parents report a neutral to moderately positive impact.

"An Attempt to Reconstruct Children's Donor Concept: A Comparison Between Children and Lesbian Parents' Attitudes Towards Donor Anonymity"
K. Vanfraussen, I. Ponjaert-Kristoffersen, and A. Brewaeys
Department of Developmental and Life Span Psychology, University of Brussels, Belgium • published in *Human Reproduction* 16:9 (2001), pp. 2,019–2,025

**Salient findings:** In general, the children wanted to know more about the donor (though their opinions were mixed), whereas the mothers preferred the donor to remain anonymous.

## SPERM BANKS

The best way to get a feel for sperm banks is to go to their Web sites and look around. I have only listed banks that offer open-identity donors. Generally, that means the donor has agreed to at least one-time contact with any offspring, should the child request it at age eighteen or older. For a broader annotated listing of sperm banks, check out www.fertilityplus.com. For names and Web sites of U.S. sperm banks go to the donor insemination links at www.choosingsinglemotherhood.com or, for a *really* comprehensive list, go to www.donorsiblingregistry.com and click "browse by clinic."

**Pacific Reproductive Services**
www.pacrepro.com

(main office)
444 DeHaro Street, Suite 222
San Francisco, CA 94107
888-469-5800
or 415-487-2288

(Pasadena office)
65 North Madison Street, Suite 610
Pasadena, CA 91101
626-432-1681
Progressive, single-mom-friendly, and run by women. Smaller operation than some, but has the largest selection of willing-to-be-known donors in the country.

**The Sperm Bank of California**
www.thespermbankofca.org
Reproductive Technologies, Inc.
2115 Milvia Street, 2nd Floor
Berkeley, CA 94704
510-841-1858
Progressive, single-mom-friendly, nonprofit sperm bank. Pioneered identity-release donors. Run by women. Informative Web site.

### Xytex Corporation
www.xytex.com
100 Emmett Street
Augusta, GA 30904-5826
800-277-3210
or 706-733-0130

One of earliest large sperm banks to offer open-identity donors. Adult photos available for some open donors. Though they don't advertise themselves as being progressive, I have heard good things about them from single moms and lesbians who have used their donors.

### California Cryobank
www.cryobank.com
11915 LaGrange Avenue
Los Angeles, CA 90025
866-927-9622
or 310-443-5244

One of the larger banks. Has started offering open-identity donors, and will contact totally anonymous donors when the children turn eighteen to see how they feel about contact.

### Fairfax Cryobank
www.fairfaxcryobank.com
3015 Williams Drive, Suite 110
Fairfax, VA 22301
800-338-8407

Another large, popular sperm bank that has recently started offering "ID consent" donors. For this bank, that means that the donor has agreed to have identifying information released, but has not necessarily agreed to a one-time meeting.

### New England Cryogenic Center, Inc.
www.necryogenic.com
153 Needham Street, Building 1
Newton, MA 02464
800-991-4999
or 617-244-4447

I had not heard of this sperm bank, but it appears to be a large one and it offers some open-identity donors.

**Rainbow Flag Health Services**

www.gayspermbank.com

510-521-7737

This is a small, single-mom-friendly sperm bank in the San Francisco Bay Area that actively recruits gay donors, though it has straight donors as well. At this bank, you will learn the identity of the donor once your child is three months old, and you are asked to contact him within the first year—sort of like open adoption. Additionally, this bank requires you to agree not to circumcise your child, a procedure that they consider genital mutilation.

### Single-Mom Support Groups

**Single Mothers by Choice**

www.singlemothersbychoice.com

P.O. Box 1642

New York, NY 10028

212-988-0993

This group, founded by Jane Mattes, author of *Single Mothers by Choice*, has thousands of members and local chapters all over the country that hold meetings and events. For a yearly membership fee, it offers access to the local groups, as well as a quarterly newsletter and active e-mail Listservs for discussion and support on every stage of the process, including thinking, trying to conceive, adopting, and parenting.

**Choosing Single Motherhood**

www.choosingsinglemotherhood.com

This is the Web site of Mikki Morrissette, author of *Choosing Single Motherhood: The Thinking Woman's Guide*. She offers a small Listserv for discussion and support, as well as free and low-fee information on issues of interest to single moms and those considering single motherhood. Good links to other relevant Web sites.

### Legal issues regarding donor insemination

**Human Rights Campaign**

www.hrc.org

1640 Rhode Island Avenue, NW

Washington, DC 20036-3278

800-777-4723

or TTY: 202-216-1572

or 202-628-4160

This is a gay-rights organization, but the site offers much information of use to straight single women considering donor insemination. Under "get informed" on their splash page, click "family" to find state by state laws on donor insemination, referrals to lawyers who will be familiar with donor insemination issues, information on choosing a sperm bank, and sample donor agreements. The site's large and a little hard to navigate, but there is a search function.

### *Fertility issues*

**Fertilityplus.com**

www.fertilityplus.com

A nonprofit fertility Web site written by patients. Good source of information on fertility issues, including how to do a home insemination.

### MAIA Midwifery & Preconception Services

www.maiamidwifery.com

23 Altarinda Road, Suite 215

Orinda, CA 94563

925-253-0685

This midwifery practice specializes in serving alternative families, including lesbian and heterosexual single moms. There are sample donor agreements on their Web site. For a fee, you can have a phone consultation in which they will go over your options, give sperm bank tips and insemination instruction, and address any questions you have about insemination or fertility.

### The American Fertility Association

www.theafa.org

305 Madison Avenue, Suite 449

New York, NY 10165

888-917-3777

This organization's Web site offers information, message boards, and referrals to doctors and therapists.

### Connecting with donor siblings and anonymous donors

**Note:** In addition to the national Donor Sibling Registry listed below, some sperm banks have their own sibling registries.

### The Donor Sibling Registry

www.donorsiblingregistry.com

This Web site, with nearly eight thousand active (paying) members, connects donor-inseminated kids with their half siblings and occasionally their donors. It also offers "success stories," where members can read about the experiences of other members who have met their biological kin, as well as relevant articles and resources and a large Listserv for discussion of donor conception issues.

### Information on doulas (professional birth attendants)

### DONA International

www.dona.org

P.O. Box 626

Jasper, IN 47547

888-788-DONA

This is the Web site of the international doula training and certification agency. You can search their huge database for a doula in your state, or learn more about what doulas do.

### DoulaWorld.com

www.doulaworld.com

Ori Eisen

6214 E. Hillery Drive

Scottsdale, AZ 85254-2568

This Web site familiarizes you with doulas, as well as offering more user-friendly information about those individual doulas in your area who have paid to be listed.

*Breast-feeding support*

**La Leche League International**
www.lalecheleague.com
This Web site has tons of information about breast-feeding, and you can also find
the phone number of a local La Leche League leader who can answer questions and
provide support.

---

### THE COSTS OF DONOR INSEMINATION

Unfortunately, it's impossible to say exactly how much donor insemination
will cost you. It depends on your fertility status, the method you use, the doctor you use, what his or her fees are and what methods he or she recommends,
the area of the country you live in (expensive versus not), which sperm bank
you use, what sort of semen you are ordering (anonymous versus open-identity,
B.A. versus Ph.D., "washed" or not), and, perhaps most of all, what your insurance covers. Some insurance plans will cover almost everything, others will
cover nothing. (Semen is never covered.) That said, here are some figures:

**Home insemination, known donor:** Free, or nearly. The cost of a syringe and
a paper cup. But this method carries legal and health risks. He could sue for
custody; you could get an STD.

**Home insemination, anonymous donor:** Between $500 and $1,300 a month,
for semen, shipping, and supplies.

**Intrauterine insemination at the doctor's office:** About $500 or more per
month. Can be several thousand. May or may not be covered by your insurance. Does not include semen.

**In vitro fertilization:** About $15,000 to $20,000 a try. May or may not be
covered by your insurance. Does not include semen.

**Anonymous donor sperm:** Between $200 and $600 a vial. Two tries (aka two
vials) a month are recommended, once the day before ovulation, once timed
to ovulation.

## FERTILITY, AGE BY AGE

Please remember that women are not statistics, that accidental pregnancies occasionally happen to women in their late forties, and that using reproductive technology can affect these numbers, which reflect women who aren't using birth control.

Women not using birth control who remained childless:

Ages 20–24    6 percent
Ages 25–29    9 percent
Ages 30–34    15 percent
Ages 35–39    30 percent
Ages 40–44    64 percent

*Source:* J. Menken, J. Trussell, and U. Larsen, "Age and Infertility," *Science* 233 (1986), pp. 1,389–1,394

## MISCARRIAGE RATES, AGE BY AGE

These are rates of miscarriage in women who had a clinical pregnancy (a gestational sac that was perceived using ultrasound).

Age 35 and under:    14 percent
Ages 35–37    19 percent
Ages 38–40    25 percent
Ages 40 and over    40 percent

*Source:* Centers for Disease Control and Prevention, Assisted Reproductive Technology Success Rates, 2001

# Index